LESS WORRY MORE LIFE

Preparing for Weight Loss Surgery:

What You Need to Know for Ultimate Success

LESS WORRY MORE LIFE

Preparing for Weight Loss Surgery:

What You Need to Know for Ultimate Success

Thomas W. Clark, MS, MD, FACS

Board Certified Bariatric Surgeon and Bariatrician

Center for Weight Loss Success, PC

LESS WORRY MORE LIFE

PREPARING FOR WEIGHT LOSS SURGERY:

WHAT YOU NEED TO KNOW FOR ULTIMATE SUCCESS

Published by Adriel Publishing

Edited by Karol H. Clark, MSN, RN

FIRST EDITION

Printed in the U.S.A.

Cover design by Liz Lawless

ISBN-10: 1-939998-02-6

ISBN-13: 978-1-939998-02-6

www.cfwls.com

Dedication

I dedicate this book to the committed individuals and their supportive fans who embrace this life changing journey of long-term weight loss and improved health. May you embark upon the journey of weight loss surgery with your eyes, minds and hearts wide open. May you experience optimal success and a fulfilling life that exceeds your expectations. Most importantly, may you enjoy your journey along the way.

I also dedicate this book to the thousands of amazing motivated people who have chosen me as their weight loss surgeon – I am honored. You and your long-term success give true meaning to what I do every day.

Finally, I dedicate this book to my parents who taught me the value of hard work, my wife and best friend who believes in me and shares my passion for excellence and to my four children who bring immense joy to my life every day.

Dr. Thomas W. Clark

Disclaimer

Some of the information in this book is anecdotal opinions from the author after practicing extensively and exclusively in the field of bariatric surgery (performing nearly 4,000 primary weight loss surgery procedures) and bariatric medicine. Unless otherwise stated, statements are based upon his extensive clinical experience (and common sense) over the past 20 years specializing in bariatric surgery and bariatric medicine. The opinions of clients are theirs and were freely given.

The information presented in this book is guidelines set forth by the author for his patients. This information is individualized for them by the author and the professional staff at the Center for Weight Loss Success based upon their particular situation.

Individual medical advice must be modified based upon the patient's individual situation by his/her chosen bariatric surgeon and primary care practitioner. The information in this book is intended to serve as a guide to people considering or undergoing weight loss surgery.

Table of Contents

For pdf downloads of the diets, menus and lists in this book along with companion videos, sign in at http://www.YourSurgeryPrep.com

A Note from the Author

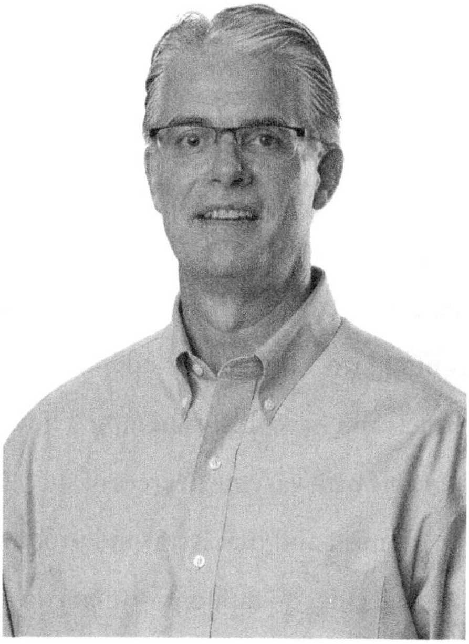

Thomas W. Clark, MS, MD, FACS

Congratulations on your decision to make healthy changes in your life through one of the most effective tools available – weight loss surgery! Congratulations also for selecting an experienced bariatric surgeon and hopefully a comprehensive weight loss surgery program that will provide you with the necessary ongoing support throughout your journey.

You have made an extremely important decision. You are planning to undergo weight loss surgery. The goal of this book is to help guide you through this life-changing event – before, during and after your surgery. Please be sure to direct specific questions to your chosen experienced bariatric surgeon. As mentioned earlier, the information presented in this book is in no way intended to replace or contradict any and all information or physician orders set forth by your chosen bariatric surgeon or primary care practitioner.

You may be experiencing various emotions at this point… from total fear of failure…to firm confidence that success will be yours this time! You have likely attempted numerous other weight loss programs with varying degrees of success. You have now invested in yourself and that is a wonderful first step.

Anyone who decides to undergo weight loss surgery is embarking on a journey. You probably have a "destination" (or goal) in mind. This destination is different for each individual (i.e. wellness, thinness, self-confidence, and improvement/elimination of various health problems).

All journeys require multiple steps. This journey is no different. Some steps are easier than others. The surgery is just a single step along the way. No two individuals' journey is the same. Please remember that it is the journey (NOT the destination) which is life itself. Your personal goals ought to include experiencing and enjoying life (the journey) to its fullest.

I have carefully written this book based on 20 years worth of experience with nearly 4,000 patients. This information is essential for long-term success. You will find this resource helpful for you and your support person(s) as you embark upon this amazing journey.

Thank you for trusting me to help you get started on your journey. I sincerely hope your efforts will bring you a fuller and healthier life, free of the disease called morbid obesity.

To receive Dr. Clark's free special report for successful weight loss, visit www.cfwls.com. You can also follow him on:

Facebook at www.facebook.com/weightlossdrclark

YouTube at www.youtube.com/docweightloss

Dr. Clark's blog at: www.cfwls.com/blog

Dr. Clark's Weekly Podcast at www.cfwls.com/podcasts

Twitter at www.twitter.com/docweightloss

Foreword

A Message Worth Reading

by Kevin Lyles

There are two things to prepare for when you finally decide to have weight loss surgery in my opinion. On one hand, there is the physical preparation. This is not as hard as it sounds. The fact is, once you set a date for your surgery you have a finite number of days to work things out physically. After that, physical things take care of themselves very quickly. The great thing about the surgery is that you will be physically unable to go off track, at least initially. You really should try to exercise some self control and practice saying no to yourself. Let's face it. The lack of this kind of discipline is what got me here in the first place.

I'm willing to bet that is true of the majority of us. We lacked the ability to effectively and consistently do push-aways, as pushing away from the dinner table. That's not a judgment. That was just a fact for me. Again, you'll see that the surgery will initially give you the discipline you've been lacking for a while.

The physical preparation, although important, is not what you need to successfully go through this surgery and the resulting lifestyle changes in my opinion. So let me tell you how I got to it and through it.

It's all about your attitude. You're saying to yourself right now, "That's just silly. I have a great attitude. I'm already a happy person. It can't be that simple." You'd be right of course. If you didn't have a great attitude it would be hard to decide to have the surgery.

The attitude that I'm speaking of is the one where you let yourself admit that there are other possibilities for you and your life than just being the "Jolly fat guy" everyone loves because you have a "great attitude". If you are looking at this surgery just to lose weight you are missing the point. I had the surgery because of my hopes. I wanted to realize the things I hoped for. That is what leads you to the second type of preparation, and maybe the most important of the two; Mental preparation.

Mental preparation starts with letting go of a lot of baggage big people carry with them every day. For instance, for me, I always worried that people were judging me by my size. I work in the financial services industry and every time I met with a client I would be thinking, "what are they thinking of me" instead of concentrating on the situation at hand. I constantly worried that my wife's or my kid's friend's were laughing at them because of their fat husband or father. I worried about having to put myself in situations that would accentuate how big I was like going to an amusement park with my kids and not fitting on rides or not being able to step down from a dock into a canoe or having to sit in a chair that everyone in the room was looking at out of the corner of their eye to see if it would actually hold me. On the tail end of all of these types of things you find that it's you judging you too. Baggage: you have to let it go and tell yourself, "I deserve better of myself and for myself.

Mentally, you have to prepare yourself for the break-up of your first love. I never thought it was true of myself, but I found that I had an emotional attachment to food. I love a great burger, a big juicy rib-eye steak, and a Chinese Buffet and I'm not ashamed to admit it. Like the song says, "Breaking up is hard to do". You have to guard against getting depressed because you can't hang out with these old tried and true friends. Friends that got you through almost every bad time in your life.

You have to be mentally tough so you will have the attitude to follow through to your goals. When you start losing so much weight after the surgery everyone will be complimentary. You have to stay strong and not buy into the "you're so skinny now, when are you going to stop" encouragement from your friends and family. You have to keep reminding yourself it's not just about weight loss. I'm changing my life and my life style. Proper attitude will help you stay focused on being healthier and letting you go do the things that add to the quality of your life. For example, as stupid as it may sound, one of my big goals (hopes) was to be able to comfortably take a trip by plane, sit in the middle seat, and not touch anyone on either side. That is not a how much you weigh thing. It's a quality of life thing. I have taken several trips since my surgery.

The flip side of having the attitude that it's okay to say yes to life and lifestyle changes is giving yourself permission to be firm and tell yourself "NO!" You have to prepare yourself not to give in to you just because it's easier to do. I love bread. It's one of my weaknesses. But, one bite of bread means I don't have the room necessary to get the amount of protein and water I need to reach my goal. So I tell myself a firm no. I have to be firm and tell myself no sitting around snacking. Get up and go to the gym. You get the picture.

You have to prepare mentally to guard against losing hope if things get tough. Concentrate on setting and working towards goals, no matter how small. I still have goals like eat at the same time, check my blood sugar, and keep track of my protein and water intake. Simple things, but they help to keep me focused.

Be prepared to know you will cheat. It will take a strong attitude towards success not to beat yourself up too much and to get back on track. Don't give up on yourself because of little setbacks. Prepare for it going in. I created a cheat sheet to get me on track. It's made up of simple things like take a walk, go to the gym, or one of my favorite things was to go to Dr. Clark's office and weigh myself. You'll only be there for a few minutes, but you'll get an unsolicited word of encouragement, see that you haven't really wrecked anything, and actually be an encouragement to someone in the program behind you.

I think the biggest preparation you can make is giving yourself permission to ask for help. The entire staff from Dr. Clark on down is here to help you succeed. Don't do what I call, "Dying from embarrassment". This is where you are too embarrassed to ask for help on simple things so you either ignore the problem, continue to do it wrong, or skip it altogether. There is nothing they won't help you with. From the great class materials to the support groups to the physical trainers they have you covered. One of my favorite proverbs is, "The teacher can open the door, but the student must walk through himself". Dr. Clark's entire staff is there to support you in whatever you need. They have it all set up. Just ask if you don't see what you're looking for.

Most important of all: You are already a SUCCESS in my book because you have taken a big step towards realizing your hopes.

Cheering for you,

Kevin Lyles

For more about Kevin's personal story, as well as his before and after photos, see Chapter 6.

Introduction

Why is education so important?

At the Center for Weight Loss Success, we have found that educated clients have the best long-term success in meeting their individual health goals. When you are educated, you are more likely to actively participate in your plan of care. You will make better decisions regarding your physical care, emotional care, diet and exercise regimen. *Education is critical to successful decision making **before** and **after** surgery.* This book focuses on the time frame before, during and after surgery. It also includes many tips for long-term success. It is intended to supplement the curriculum provided by your chosen surgeon as an additional tool for your weight loss success.

Everyone's health goals are different. You should use this guide and individualize it for your specific needs.

You can do it!

How do I get the most out of this curriculum?

This curriculum is a "guide". Please note that everyone's experiences are slightly different but these guidelines have been developed over 20 years of supporting individuals just like you through their journey following weight loss surgery. ***However, this curriculum is not intended to take the place of personal discussions with your surgeon or one of his/her expert staff members.***

To get the most out of this curriculum, **please read all the information provided.** It is intended to be a resource to you and your support person(s). **Refer to it often.**

Chapter 1 Identifies common medical problems associated with obesity.

Chapter 2 Addresses the many psychological/behavioral changes that are associated with weight loss surgery. You should not ignore this very important aspect of your care. Your emotional health and overall attitude and commitment can make the difference in your long-term success and how you cope with the many changes associated with weight loss surgery.

Chapter 3 Addresses your preparation for surgery, your surgical experience and your post-operative care and follow-up.

Chapter 4 Outlines specific recommended dietary guidelines to follow **prior** to your surgery. We recommend you follow one of the two suggested diets in this chapter for two weeks prior to your surgery. This is recommended in order to jump-start your weight loss and decrease the potential risks while undergoing weight loss surgery.

Chapter 5 Addresses the common dietary changes you must follow **after** your weight loss surgery. It provides a guide for your daily intake as you progress from a liquid diet, to a blenderized diet, and beyond to "real food". This section also addresses vitamins, supplements, reading labels, alcohol, and many other topics. You will find a pre-operative "shopping list" to utilize as you prepare for surgery.

Chapter 6 Is critical to your success and addresses the importance of exercise. You will find your weight loss progress will not be as successful if exercise is not included as a part of your daily habits. During weight loss, it is extremely important to maintain and build lean body mass (and subsequently increase your metabolic rate). Loss of lean body mass will slow your metabolism, slow your weight loss, and make it much easier to regain weight.

Chapter 7 Includes a review of the weight loss surgery procedures. These procedures give you the "tool" to assist you in losing weight. In addition, the procedural risks and typical results and outcomes are identified.

Chapter 8 The last section Includes supplemental bonus information for your long-term success. This section may be the most important one of this entire curriculum. You will find an easy to use action list and information reviewing the optimal use of your gastric pouch/tool for weight loss and long-term weight control. In addition, information regarding what you can do prior to surgery is listed along with references, helpful resources and informative websites.

Weight Loss Surgery – "A Life-Changing Event"

Working with you as you undergo weight loss surgery is truly rewarding. I have the opportunity and honor to witness wonderful, fun, intelligent people becoming transformed over time. You remain the same wonderful, fun, intelligent person within a new healthier self. The weight loss enhances your ability to do things you may not have been able to do before or in a long time. Hearing you share that you can "cross your legs", "become a firefighter again", "play with my children/grandchildren", "walk over a mile", "go back to work" or "walk without a cane anymore" is truly amazing. It is these "non-measurable" outcomes that make it all worthwhile. In addition, the measurable outcomes (lower blood pressure, elimination of diabetes, improved joint pain, etc…) are just as rewarding.

Weight loss surgery is a life-changing event that involves hard work, commitment, support, and occasional discomfort. I can't do the work for you, but I can support you and educate you along the way. I can share in your successes and frustrations. You will begin a new eating pattern that will **never** be the same. You will make sacrifices, but with perseverance, a positive attitude and a life of good choices, you will use your new tool effectively and share in your own successes.

Weight Loss Surgery as a Tool

Weight loss surgery decreases the current size of your stomach (approximately 2 liters) to a few ounces. This new pouch or "tool" decreases the amount of food you are able to ingest. Like any tool, it can be used correctly or incorrectly.

Initially (during first 1-3 months) you will likely have little or no hunger. It is easier during this time to follow the prescribed diet. However, over time, if the "tool" is used incorrectly (such as drinking high calorie liquids) you will have relatively poor weight loss or even weight gain over a period of time. **It is still diet, exercise and behavior change which produces weight loss.**

With the proper use of this book and the education provided by your surgeon and his/her expert team, you will have the information necessary to use your new small stomach properly and effectively. This will assist you in attaining long-term weight loss and realization of your health goals. ***Remember that bariatric surgeons all have slightly different recommendations for their patients. This book is in no way intended to replace his/her recommendations.***

CHAPTER 1

Obesity

Health Consequences of Obesity

As you are likely aware, there are many health consequences of obesity. A summary of health consequences are identified below. It is important to note that more than 300,000 deaths per year are attributed to the health consequences of obesity1. In fact, only cigarette smoking is the cause of more preventable deaths in the United States.

Health Consequences of Obesity

Respiratory System

- Shortness of Breath & fatigue
- Obstructive sleep apnea
- Hypoventilation syndrome

Endocrine System

- Reduced insulin sensitivity
- Glucose intolerance
- Diabetes mellitus-Type II
- Dyslipidemia

Cardiovascular System

- Hypertension/High blood pressure
- Congestive heart failure
- Varicose veins
- Pulmonary embolism
- Coronary artery disease

Musculoskeletal System

- Immobility
- Degenerative arthritis
- Low back pain
- Accident proneness

Circulatory

- Venous stasis of legs
- Cellulitis
- Diminished hygiene
- Skin infections

Female Health Issues

- Urinary stress incontinence
- Infertility
- Absence of menstruation
- Breast and uterine cancer
- Menstrual irregularities

Gastrointestinal

- Reflux esophagitis
- Hepatic steatosis
- Gallbladder disease
- Hernias
- Colon cancer

Psychosocial

- Work disability
- Social discrimination
- Depression

If you suffer from any of these health consequences, you know how negatively they affect your finances and your overall ability to function in the workforce and at home. Helping people just like you reverse/cure such health problems is very rewarding. As an example, I see about 85% of my patients with Type II diabetes eliminate their need for supplemental diabetic medications within 1-2 weeks after surgery. Of course, there is no guarantee but the statistics are staggering.

Steve Clemmons Testimonial
(lost 200 pounds)

I've struggled with my weight my whole life, losing it only to regain double the amount I lost. I had given up on the thought of being healthy. My first eye opener was a denial of additional life insurance. My wife and I were Foster Parents and about to adopt 2 children we had in our home. Shortly after, when my yearly physical results showed diabetes, high blood pressure and borderline cholesterol numbers, my doctor suggested weight loss surgery. He told me, the statistics proved my weight coupled with the diabetes and hypertension would shorten my life.

I still struggled with the decision at first, but my family supported me and after talking with Dr Clark and his staff, I was confident and hopeful. It has been one year and I have lost an astounding 200 pounds, and 20 inches from my waist. I feel like a new man with more energy than ever! Also, my clothes fit better and I'm no longer hot all the time.

All of my health indicators such as laboratory tests and my BMI have greatly improved. Best yet, I no longer have to take medication! All along I've received awesome support from the Center for Weight Loss Success, Dr. Clark and his experienced staff. They all truly care about their patients and strive to provide you the information required for success.

Before

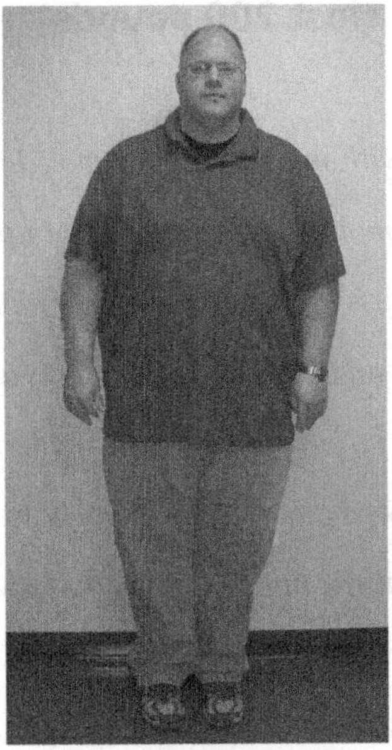

After

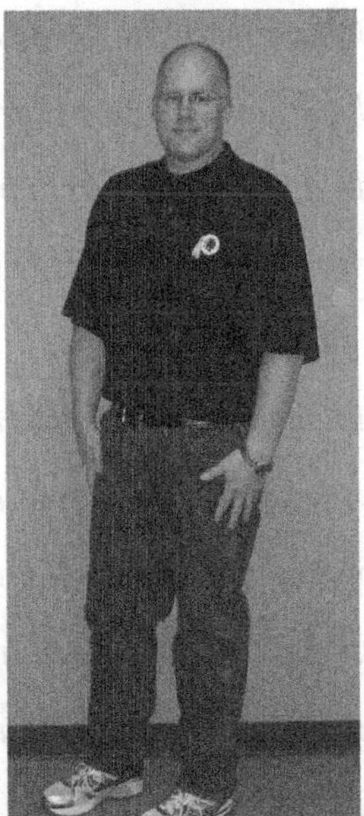

CHAPTER 2

Behavioral/Habit Modification

Psychology and Weight Loss Surgery

Emotions play into why you gain weight. Emotions also affect your ability to lose weight and keep it off long-term. Weight loss surgery is a tool to lose weight, but unless you change some of your underlying habits related to nutrition and activity, you will be less likely to experience long-term success. You **must** be able to commit to these changes.

As a part of your weight loss program, you may have **week-**

ly Behavior Modification classes. These are usually special and designed for you and others like you who have committed to a long-term answer to overcoming obesity. If offered by your surgeon, participation in these classes will not only provide you with additional support, they will provide you with what you need to replace your unhealthy habits with healthy ones. These new habits will gradually become ones you can live with for life.

Having surgery does not mean that you need to feel deprived for the rest of your life. Surgery is a part of your overall plan to change your diet, activity and habits. You will turn unhealthy behaviors into an easy to implement lifestyle of improved health and vitality. You are not alone and the choice(s) are yours...let us help you determine what **you "can" do** to succeed instead of focusing on what you "can't" do.

Some topics that require attention before and after surgery include:

Emotional Well Being

As you lose weight, your emotional well-being is very important. We want you to be able to identify coping mechanisms prior to surgery. These tools need to be readily available after surgery. We also would like to warn you of some of the feelings you may have after surgery (i.e. vulnerability, anxiety, and depression). These feelings may occur and are normal. Understand that it is "ok" to ask for help from your current mental health professional or our clinical psychologist. Assistance is not required by everyone but can be an integral part to your overall care.

Anxiety

Anxiety is a feeling experienced by everyone. We generally become anxious when we experience change. Since weight loss surgery is a "life-changing event", it is normal to experience some degree of anxiety. (In fact, we worry more if a person appears to have no anxiety at all.) Anxiety becomes a hindrance if it affects your ability to perform everyday functions either before or after surgery. It is a good idea to verbalize your anxieties. In addition, it helps to become an active member of your support group before surgery so you can discuss your feelings with someone who has been through the experience of weight loss surgery. If you desire, an appointment with a licensed clinical psychologist can usually be arranged via a referral from your experienced bariatric surgeon.

Depression

Many (or even most) overweight individuals have experienced or are experiencing some degree of depression. This does not prohibit them from having surgery but serious clinical depression must be under control prior to surgery. It is also not uncommon for individuals to become depressed **after** surgery. You encounter so many changes as you progress throughout your journey that depression can occur. It is important to identify signs and symptoms of depression so that, if necessary, counseling can be arranged.

Signs of depression include extreme fatigue, mood swings, loss of interest in activities, overeating, and anger to name a few. Depression can be dangerous. It requires intervention when it affects a person's ability to perform basic activities of daily living (getting out of bed, personal hygiene, getting dressed, and getting out of the house or bedroom) or if a person feels the desire to hurt themselves or others. In these cases, the person requires immediate professional intervention.

We mention these potential causes of depression so that you can be aware of them. This does not mean that you will experience any or all of them. We just want you to be aware of these potential causes of depression so you can identify them if they happen to you. You can then anticipate their possibility of occurring, and have a **plan/coping mechanism** in place if necessary.

Body Image

Your perception of your body image is a hard thing to change. After surgery, clients often cannot visualize themselves as being any different than prior to surgery. It is common for clients to tell us that they can walk by a window or mirror and *"don't know who the person is staring back at them"*. Although they may have lost at least 100 pounds, they still visualize themselves as morbidly obese. They also find it hard to shop for appropriate sizes – still migrating toward the "plus" sizes even though they no longer wear that size. Time and a positive attitude will help you embrace these positive image changes.

Emotional Eating

Food has likely been an important part of your life. Some refer to food as being *"my best friend - something that was always there to help me cope with stress"*. Like many humans, you probably use food to cope with many personal feelings and social situations (celebrations, holidays, boredom, anger, anxiety, fear, sadness etc…). Dealing with the emotional bond you have with food will be one of the hardest to overcome. It is important to begin to deal with these feelings **prior** to surgery rather than after surgery. We will be discussing new coping mechanisms (instead of emotional eating) later in this chapter.

Some clients cope with this feeling by having many "last

suppers" prior to surgery. We strongly discourage this. We would prefer you actually begin the habit of healthy eating prior to surgery and focus on getting into your best physical health now rather than later. Weight loss surgery is a major operation and morbidly obese clients have increased risk factors. If you can lose some weight prior to surgery, this would definitely be a step in the right direction. Although we do not currently **require** weight loss prior to surgery (like some surgeons do) it is strongly recommended and supported (see Section 4 for further discussion).

Common Feelings Prior to Surgery

It is common to experience a flood of various feelings prior to surgery. We review these common emotions to help reassure you that these are normal. In addition, we share ways to cope with some of the feelings.

Excitement

You have made a decision to embark upon a life-changing journey. You are making a commitment to a lifetime of healthier activities (diet and exercise) and you anticipate the positive effects it will likely have on your life. It is good to be excited about surgery. Share your joy with others (as you choose to) and celebrate your healthy decision.

Anxiety

You realize that this surgery has risks. You have determined that the benefits outweigh the risks and you are ready to proceed. This is a decision only you can make. Anxiety remains related to the procedure, the potential effects it will have on your life and how you will adapt. Your surgeon and his/her expert team will help support you and provide you with guidance to help maintain your anxiety at a healthy level. Please ask your surgeon if you have any questions. Your surgeon and his/her team are there for your support as you make your new journey.

Fear

Many clients express fear related to many factors. Some are physical - such as the surgery itself, potential pain, potential complications and dietary changes. Some factors are emotional - such as "*Who should I tell and when?*", "*Will my family and friends be supportive?*" and "*What if I fail?*" These are all very common. How you cope with fear is very individualized. Some rely on their spiritual beliefs and prayer. Some talk to other clients or healthcare professionals regarding their questions and fears. Your surgeon and his/her team will encourage you to become as educated as possible regarding the surgery and use healthy, adaptive coping skills.

Shame/Guilt

Some clients express feelings of shame and guilt regarding weight loss surgery. They feel they are taking "the easy way out" or that they are such a failure that this is a "last resort". Weight loss surgery IS NOT "the easy way out" nor a "last resort" for weight loss. Weight loss surgery provides obese clients with a long-term weight loss solution that requires commitment and a great deal of work and sacrifice. You can be proud of yourself as you begin and continue through your journey toward a new you.

Confidence

Confidence is a beautiful attribute. You have control of your destiny. You are taking a giant step toward meeting your health goals. You have researched your options and made a decision to have weight loss surgery. You deserve success. Confidence will help guide you toward your goals. Confidence will keep you enjoying the journey (which is life itself) along the way.

Stress Management

Like depression, stress is harmful to the body as well as the mind. Not only is surgery a stressor, but the changes associated with this event are stressful as well. It is important to think through potential stressors in your life and develop realistic coping mechanisms.

Do this **prior** to surgery so that these coping mechanisms are readily available for implementation when necessary.

Stress – What is it?

Stress is your reaction to an actual or potential threat. A stress response starts in the brain which sends signaling hormones and nerve impulses to the rest of the body to prepare for "fight or flight". Your body is readying itself to deal with the change. This is normal and natural. When confronting a threat, the adrenal glands release epinephrine (adrenaline), which makes the heart pump faster and the lungs work harder to flood the body with oxygen. The adrenal glands also release extra cortisol and other glucocorticoids, which help the body convert sugars into energy. Nerve cells also release norepinephrine, which tenses the muscles and sharpens the senses to prepare for action. Finally, digestion shuts down in preparation to flee or fight.

As noted earlier, this is your body's normal reaction. However, your body is also supposed to have a "calming down" period following the "fight or flight" period. Too often we do not allow our bodies the recovery time it needs. You would not drive your car 70 miles an hour, 24 hours a day, 7 days a week because it would break down. However, we do the equivalent to our bodies without giving it a second thought - until we break down. Instead of allowing our body to recover, we let it recover only a little. Then we are back facing another stressor. These stressors tend to build and build until you reach a breaking point. At this point you usually get upset about something that is not even that important. The real reason you are getting upset is because you did not manage your stress effectively.

The influx of hormones to your body during the "fight or flight" stage can be very damaging short-term as well as long-term. "When the threat passes, epinephrine and norepinephrine levels drop, but if danger comes too often they can damage the arteries. Chronic low level stress keeps the glucocorticoids in circulation, leading to a weakened immune system, loss of bone mass, suppression of the reproductive system and memory problems2." Thus, long-term effects of stress include a weakened immune system, damaged cardiovascular system and damaged/weakened bones.

Stress is alive and well in everyone's life. It is imperative to learn what causes stress in your life and try to deal with these factors. For some situations, you may be able to avoid the factors, for others, you must begin to develop lifelong coping mechanisms for dealing with them and their negative side effects.

Ways to Manage Stress

You can manage stress through the use of coping skills. These skills can be used on either a "preventive" level (utilizing coping skills on a daily basis to keep your baseline stress level low) or by "catching it" when you feel the beginning signs of stress and using your coping skills at that time.

Developing and practicing realistic coping skills that work for you are very important. Think about what will work for you. Some coping skills commonly utilized include:

- Exercise
- Reading
- Talking with someone
- Crafts
- Hobbies
- Spirituality/Prayer
- Deep Breathing
- Meditation

Taking Care of Yourself FIRST

Most people (especially women) spend so much time taking care of others, they rarely take time for themselves. Unfortunately, if you don't take care of yourself, you may not be as effective or able to care for others. **Taking care of yourself is not selfish,** it is critical to your mental and physical well being.

Jean Midyette, MSA, BSN, RNC-MNN Testimonial (lost 130 pounds)

I was a skinny child and adolescent, particularly the year that I grew 6 inches in my sophomore year of high school. I was a slender young adult through nursing school and only began to experience difficulties keeping my weight within normal limits after my third pregnancy. I began a series of diets where I would lose up to fifty pounds only to put it back on again. I went on not one but two full liquid, medically supervised fasts and always gained the weight back.

My weight continued to increase over the years until I found on one family trip that I had great difficulty fitting into an airline seat and could not fasten the seat belt. I felt so terrible that I did not ask the flight attendant for help I just threw a sweater over my stomach and tried to act relaxed as if I were buckled up. I felt so terrible and worried that a bumpy flight would jerk me out of my seat and put me on the floor of the plane. I knew I needed to do something about my increasing weight, increasing blood pressure and declining health but felt I didn't have the energy or power to do anything about it.

My personal physician suggested that I have weight loss surgery but I was afraid of complications of surgery and the malabsorption of nutrients and other issues associated with weight loss surgery. This suggestion did make me start thinking about weight loss surgery. I went on a crash diet and lost almost 75 pounds all by myself.

I stopped weighing myself and rapidly gained the weight back and more. Every time I went to the doctor I refused to be weighed. I simply did not want to see the evidence of my out of control eating. I hated to be hungry and I ate when I was stressed. Eating was soothing and food was my drug of choice. When my primary care physician had to put me on a third blood pressure medication I knew I had to lose the weight. But how would I do it? I always gained the weight back and more.

I had heard some colleagues discussing alternatives to traditional weight loss surgery and asked them some questions about it. I asked who had done their procedures and how much weight they had lost. I began to think about the new weight loss surgery techniques and how they might work for me. When I was working at a local hospital I knew of Dr. Clark and his excellent reputation as a surgeon and decided to go to an information session at his office to learn more about the latest techniques in weight loss surgery.

I made an appointment to attend the information session at Dr. Clark's office. Dr. Clark explained the three weight loss procedures which he performed, in detail, with all of the potential complications as well as all of the benefits. I knew right away that this was the help that I needed to be successful in my weight loss.

I began my weight loss and healthy lifestyle journey on April 23, 2012 when I had the outpatient gastric sleeve procedure. One year later, I have lost 130 pounds. and haven't looked back! I have so much energy and feel so good that I started a second Master's degree program. I am on schedule to complete my Master of Science in Nursing Education in the summer of 2014. I work full time and am leading an active lifestyle. My husband and I took a 14 day trip to the Holy Land and I even lost 8 pounds on the trip. I never would have been able to enjoy our trip without having lost my weight because we did so much walking and didn't slow down the entire trip.

Dr. Clark and his staff are so supportive and always there if you need them. You can go to the office for support groups and meetings or you can get your education on line as I do. I have even downloaded the Center for Weight Loss Success cookbook from the web site. What is missing from so many weight loss programs is adequate preparation, ongoing and long term support. The Center for Weight Loss Success, Dr. Clark and his wonderful and caring staff are only a phone call or visit away. I am thrilled with the results of my weight loss and am much healthier and more active. Thank you Dr. Clark and thank you to the staff at the Center for Weight Loss Success!

BEFORE

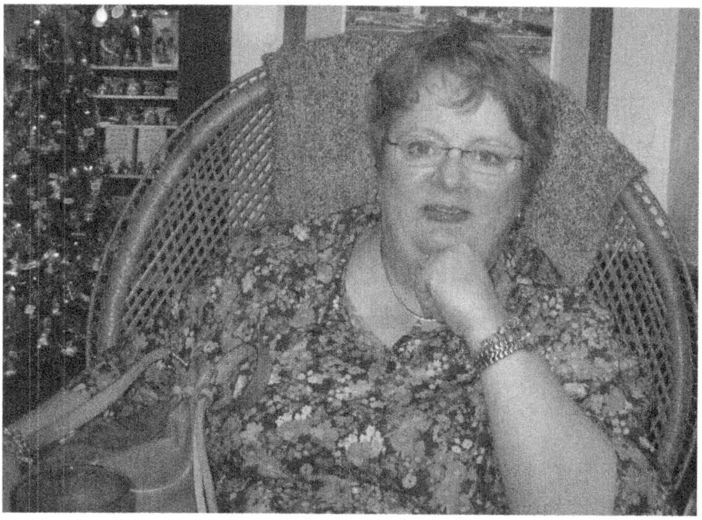

AFTER

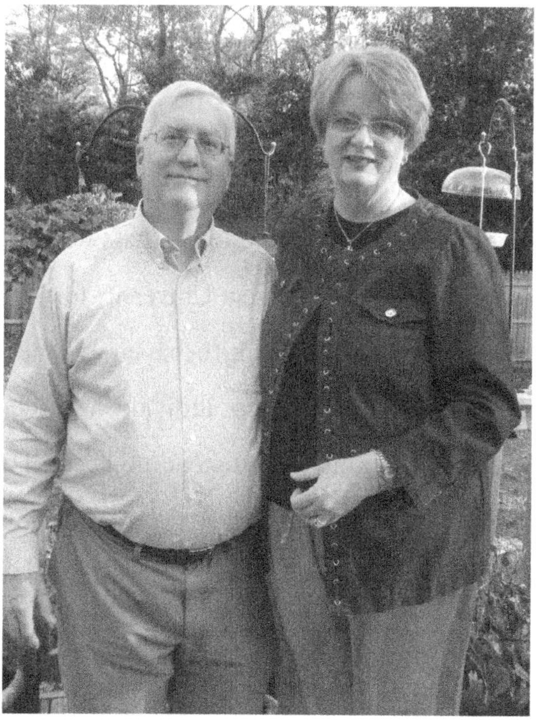

CHAPTER 3

The Surgery Experience

As you know by now, surgery is a tool but it is what you do with your new tool that creates results. That's why full participation in your Weight Management University for Weight Loss Surgery™ program is so important (behavior & fitness classes, webinars, monthly support group, individualized counseling, physician visits, monthly newsletters/modules/CD's/DVD's, personal training and more). This exclusive comprehensive program was designed with you and your optimal results in mind so really make the most of it. You have an exciting journey ahead of you and the bottom line is – we want you to be successful! If you are not a patient at the Center for Weight Loss Success, active participation in the program provided by your surgeon is critical! It was also designed with you in mind and will reinforce the information you need to know before and after surgery.

Weight loss surgery is an important decision and it can be easy to get overwhelmed. The purpose of this chapter is to guide you from your pre-operative phase to the first few months after surgery so your journey is mapped out and easy to follow. Be sure to follow your appointment schedule which keeps you on track for optimal success. You should never leave your surgeon's office without clearly understanding what your next step is and when your next visit, counseling session, personal training or group class appointment is scheduled.

Preparing for Surgery

Wish List

Often people view surgery from a number perspective (i.e. how many pounds they would like to lose). Weight loss surgery is about so much more than that. It is about enabling yourself to accomplish things that might not have been possible in the past. It is about having an exciting life. A life you can experience to the fullest extent. It is very important to think about (and document) life goals related to your weight loss. Then you can celebrate the positive changes transforming your life. Some of the "dreams" that people have shared include:

- Walking up the stairs or to the corner of their street without getting short of breath
- Playing with their children or grandchildren
- Crossing their legs
- Painting their toenails
- Stop worrying about being able to fit into a chair at a public place or worrying that it will break when they sit on it
- Fitting in a bathtub and having water on both sides
- Shopping in a store for regular sized people
- Riding a bicycle
- Returning to a productive lifestyle
- Stop worrying about going to a restaurant that might only have booths or chairs with arms on them
- Going to a movie and fitting into the seat

Take some time to identify your "wish list" and document it. After surgery, review your particular list and celebrate your progress. Check them off as you accomplish the "impossible". Look at these items as a personal challenge and celebrate all you have earned and accomplished.

Getting Your Mind and Body Ready

In the weeks or days before surgery, you need to consider yourself in training. Just as athletes prepare for a race, you can prepare yourself to be in top form for surgery. When you actively get your body and mind ready you likely will:

- Have fewer complications from anesthesia and surgery
- Be able to cooperate with necessary treatments
- Heal faster and feel better quicker
- Have better control of your pain

There are some very specific things you need to do to be in the best shape possible. You need to begin these things NOW. We know that the very worst time to try to learn things is right after surgery when you may feel foggy from anesthesia and uncomfortable from your operation. Learn and practice these things NOW so that you will be able to help yourself after surgery.

Focus on healthy eating. The better nourished you are, the more quickly your tissues will heal. Healing is WORK for your body. Good nutrition helps you tolerate the stresses on your body and to offset limits on food and fluids right after surgery. Weight loss prior to your surgery can decrease your risk and improve recovery time after surgery.

If you are a smoker – QUIT! This is easier said than done, but even a few weeks of not smoking increases the safety of anesthesia. You will not be allowed to smoke while hospitalized because you will need all your oxygen for healing. If you need help, engage the assistance of your primary care provider.

Build your exercise tolerance. Toning your muscles and building your strength will help you bounce back quicker. Walking is a perfect exercise for you prior to surgery. It is normal to feel a little weak after surgery, but you can reduce this by toning up with daily exercise.

Exercise your lungs! Practice your deep breathing. After surgery you will be encouraged to do this. Expanding your lungs helps your system get rid of anesthesia drugs quickly, helps prevent pneumonia, and speeds oxygen to your tissues to help you heal quickly. You will also FEEL better.

Move your legs to prevent blood clots!!!! After an operation, the best exercise to help your circulation and reduce your chance of blood clots will be walking! The nurses in the hospital will get you up after a brief recovery period following surgery. Once you go home, you should rest as needed but also get up and walk around as much as you can tolerate. You can do these exercises in bed or sitting in a chair during any rest periods.

1. Lying on your back in bed, "walk" your feet toward your body until your knees are fully bent. Tighten your abdominal muscles while you do this. Now let your legs slide gently back

to the flat position and repeat this four more times.

2. Lying in bed or sitting up, point your toes as if you were trying to bend your foot backwards. Hold for the count of five and relax. You should feel a "pull" on the muscles in the front of your legs. Next point your heels away from your body, tightening your leg muscles. Hold for the count of five and relax. You should feel this pull in the back of your legs. Repeat the pointing exercises 5-10 times.

Your Mind and Spirit

Now that you have decided to have surgery, **focus your mind on a good outcome.** You are the most important player in this team effort, and much will depend on your ability to fully participate. Your feelings and thoughts will play a very big part in your recovery. Reassure yourself that the best people, equipment and techniques are supporting you during surgery.

Use the power of your relationships to gather a support group. Enlist family and friends to help you keep your spirits up. Let friends and neighbors help with chores and meals. We all do better when we know we are supported by people who care about us and are cheering us on. Don't underestimate the power of your emotions. Positive thinking is the biggest help you can give yourself. Think hopeful, optimistic thoughts about the experience ahead, and start NOW!

Your Pre-Operative Plan

By the time you are reading this book (and prior to surgery), you should have accomplished the following:

- Free weight loss surgery seminar and/or completion of an informational webinar with your surgeon
- One-on-one physician consultation with your surgeon
- Pre-Operative Education Class (or whatever pre-opera tive educational program your surgeon offers)
- Be working on your pre-operative weight loss plan as prescribed/recommended by your surgeon
- Consider beginning attending the weekly Behavior Modification Classes/Webinars as available with your bariatric surgeon and his/her expert staff
- Completed any required pre-operative clearances as appropriate based upon your medical history as determined by your bariatric surgeon
- Attended or have scheduled your pre-operative testing at the hospital. These tests will be ordered by your bariatric surgeon and are required and mandated by the anesthesia staff at the hospital to give an overall picture of your health and baseline data. Your surgeon will usually review these results with you at your pre-operative visit prior to surgery.

Check with your surgeon but he/she will likely have you stop taking any medications that can potentially act as blood

thinners at least 7-10 days prior to surgery. This includes aspirin, NSAID's (i.e. Advil, Nuprin, Motrin etc.), EFA's or fish oils and some herbal supplements such as ginkgo or garlic.

Your Pre-Operative Visit with Your Surgeon

The purpose of your pre-operative visit (usually the week prior to your scheduled surgery) is for your surgeon to take time with you and your family to focus on any other questions you may have prior to surgery. Education is extremely important so you will likely hear him/her discuss much of the information already reviewed in the seminar, educational class and outlined in this handbook. A general overview of this important visit includes the following actions by your surgeon. He/she will likely:

- Take the time to answer any other questions you or your family may have
- Review your pre-operative test results
- Review your past medical/surgical history and current medications
- Complete a brief physical/check your temperature, blood pressure, pulse and respirations
- Review what to expect the day before surgery
- Inform you what time to be at the hospital and where to report

- Review what to expect the day of surgery
- Witness you sign your hospital and office consents as appropriate (the process/timing for signing consents will vary based upon surgeon protocol).

The Day Before Surgery

Try not to be over-scheduled the day before surgery. In addition, you should get a good night's sleep so you are well rested prior to surgery. Some of the surgeries are out-patient so you do not need to pack much for the hospital. In fact, the less the better. Please leave your jewelry and valuables at home for safe keeping. If you are expecting to stay overnight, you may want to bring:

- A warm robe (even in the summer, hospitals can be cold)
- Slip-proof slippers that are easy to put on
- Several pairs of socks
- Your own toiletries, toothbrush & toothpaste, comb, brush, deodorant and lotion

It is a good idea to take a thorough bath or shower and wash your hair the night before surgery. Remove all makeup and nail polish.

The day before surgery your surgeon will let you know what you may/may not eat or drink. As a general rule, I usu-

ally have you stay on liquids only such as Jell-O, clear broth, non-citrus juices, soda, coffee and tea. You may continue the use of high quality/approved protein shakes if you have already started them.

Your surgeon will give you specific orders but generally, after midnight on the night before your surgery, you are not allowed to have anything to eat or drink EXCEPT your regular medicines on the morning of surgery as instructed by your surgeon with just a sip of water.

The Day of Surgery and Post-Operative Hospital Stay

Please note that this entire chapter includes general guidelines. You must refer to the orders set forth by your bariatric surgeon and his/her expert team. If you are having surgery at the Center for Weight Loss Success, your ongoing education and Weight Management University for Weight Loss Surgery™ program will be guiding you through this process each step of the way.

On the morning of surgery, you will usually be instructed to go to the hospital at least two hours prior to your scheduled surgery. You will be interviewed by a nurse about your past medical history, the medicines you take, allergies to medicine or food, and any needs or concerns you have. Your blood pressure and temperature will be taken. You will probably be asked the same questions several times by different people. Be patient, these questions are repeated so that everyone who takes care of you will be aware of your needs. A doctor or nurse from the anesthesia department will also usually speak with you to discuss your anesthetic.

Before you go to the operating room (OR), an IV will be started. IV's let us give you the fluids and medicines you need during surgery. The hospital nurse can tell your family where to wait. Encourage your family to take reading materials along. Although the actual surgery may not be too long, the getting ready time and the recovery time can make for a long wait.

Before you go to the OR, you will be asked to remove your underwear, jewelry, and hair accessories and empty your bladder. You will change into a hospital gown. You may be given medication to dry out your mouth and relax your muscles. Your vision may get blurry and you may feel drowsy. This is normal! If you use eyeglasses, a hearing aid or dentures, leave them with your family.

FINALLY, you will be taken to the operating room, a brightly lit, busy, and sometimes noisy room. Everyone but you will wear a mask. The nurses will help you to the operating bed and place a safety belt across you. The operating room staff will help you position your arms to prevent them from sliding off the table during surgery. The anesthetist will connect you to a heart monitor which you will hear beeping. An automatic blood pressure cuff will tighten frequently to keep track of how you are doing. You will probably have an oxygen mask lightly over your nose and mouth. Breathe deeply. The medicine that puts you to sleep is given in the IV and may feel cold. Thanks to our modern drugs going to sleep is usually a gradual, pleasant experience. Focus on good, happy thoughts as you drift to sleep.

After you are asleep, the anesthetist will place an airway tube in your mouth. This keeps your throat open so that oxygen reaches your lungs. You will be positioned and special elastic "anti-clot" stockings will be placed on your legs if that has not been done already. The area where the incision(s) are made will usually be cleansed and shaved. You may not be aware of any of this. When the surgery is over and you are in the recovery room, your surgeon will talk with your family.

After the Operation

You will probably wake up in the recovery room. If you are in pain, tell the nurse. You will be sleepy and confused until the anesthetic medications wear off. Try to relax and sleep if you can.

Depending upon what type of surgery you are having, you

may have the following *temporary* things:

- One or more IV lines in your arms to supply fluids
- An oxygen mask or cannula
- Wound drains or "grenades" that remove body fluids

that collect after the operation. These will help reduce the chances of swelling or infections. The fluid will be pink or red at first. This is normal.

- A dressing covering any incisions/puncture wounds uti lized to perform the procedure

These items have a specific purpose and will be removed as soon as possible so we ask you to be patient with them. When you are awake enough, you will be transferred to the nursing unit.

Postoperative Period – The Day of Surgery

If your surgery is an outpatient procedure, you will go back to the pre-operative area once you are recovering from the anesthetic. Your family can sit with you once you leave the recovery room. You will likely undergo an Upper GI study prior to going home later that day. If you are spending the night at the hospital, you will be transferred from the recovery room to a hospital room.

During your post-operative period, the nurse will perform a clinical assessment of how you are doing. He/she will check your vital signs (BP, temperature, pulse, respirations) and orient you and your family to your room (bed, call light to contact a nurse, lights, and any necessary medical equipment). He/she will also check any tubes you have in place (IV/fluids and wound drains). They will also check your dressings on your incision and make sure the special leg hose are on your legs as well as a device called an SCD (sequential compression device). These measures help prevent clots while you are less active immediately after surgery.

The nurse will review the importance of coughing/deep breathing and the use of an incentive spirometer to help ensure your lungs are expanded. This helps to prevent the development of fluid in your lungs and the possibility of pneumonia. Coughing will be less painful if you "splint" your upper abdomen by supporting the area firmly with a pillow.

The nurse will assist you out of bed. They will help you sit at the side of the bed or in a chair. At first you may need someone to help you get up and down. Changing positions may make you uncomfortable and tired, but your strength will increase and the pain will decrease. Remember that returning to activity helps you get your strength back and also helps prevent complications.

You may be thirsty. You will be allowed to have ice chips. Once the UGI test is completed and "ok'd" you will usually be allowed to start sipping on liquids and the protein drinks. Drinking and eating before your body is ready is dangerous. For your safety and comfort, make sure that you go **very slowly** with the ice chips and sips of liquids.

Postoperative Day #1 (for those staying in the hospital)

Be sure to call for assistance if you feel dizzy or lightheaded when you attempt to get out of bed. The nurse will assist you so you can get up and use the restroom for urination. A care coordinator from the hospital may meet with you (generally on postoperative day #1). An upper GI study is obtained on this day (if it wasn't done the day of surgery) and once it is "Ok'd", you may start sipping on your liquid diet (protein supplements). You will likely be going home this afternoon. Any drains will usually be removed prior to you going home.

For anyone who has had an open procedure, your nurse may remove your abdominal dressing and clean your incision. Don't be afraid to look at your incision. Most patients are pleasantly surprised to discover how clean the area looks. You will probably have absorbable stitches. Most patients are allowed to shower the day after surgery. If you are allowed to shower you may let water run on the area but don't scrub the area. Pat it dry gently.

Postoperative Day #2

At home, it is important to continue to ambulate/walk at least 4-6 times a day and continue your coughing/deep breathing and use of your spirometer.

Going Home/Discharge Instructions *(Once again, these are general guidelines utilized at the Center for Weight Loss Success. Please refer to the specific discharge instructions set forth by your bariatric surgeon.):*

Essentially you can go home when:

- You can tolerate liquids
- You can control your pain with oral pain medication

At this point, you can recuperate as well at home as you can in the hospital (perhaps better). Your nurse will take time to review the following discharge instructions prior to your leaving the hospital.

Diet:

Continue with liquid diet until you are seen at the office. Make sure to stay hydrated and continue **to sip** all day. Your protein goal is 80-100 grams of protein each day. Please review the liquid diet instructions on pages 40-42.

Activity:

- Walking is encouraged but rest when you get tired.
- You may take a shower.

- You may climb stairs (take your time).
- No lifting more than 20 pounds for the first 2 weeks.
- If it is hurting you to do it, then you probably shouldn't be doing it yet.
- DO NOT drive for 3-4 days. You may drive when com fortable after that.

Wound Care:

- Clean incisions with soapy water when in the shower.
- Leave on steri-strips until they fall off.
- A small amount of drainage may be present from the incisions. Contact the office for any increase in drainage or associated fever >100.5.

Medications:

- You likely received a prescription for a pain medication at your pre-operative visit or prior to discharge from the hospital. If you need it, take it. If you don't need it, don't take it.
- You likely also received a prescription for an antacid medication (to prevent ulcers while you are healing). This should be taken 2 times per day for the first two months. These medications are usually Zantac, Pepcid, Prilosec or Prevacid. It is fine to use over the counter things such as Maalox, Mylanta, Pepto Bismal for any stomach upset.
- It is generally ok to take Tylenol unless you are allergic

to it.

- Arthritis medications such as Advil, Motrin, Naprosyn, or other similar drugs should be avoided.
- It is generally fine to restart other arthritis medications if needed as long as they are not upsetting your small stomach. Remember a little irritation in a tiny stomach can be a lot of irritation.
- Take a chewable multivitamin twice a day.
- Over the counter medications are usually fine as long as they are not irritating your small stomach.
- Milk of Magnesia will help with any constipation.
- It is fine to take your usual home medications. Blood pressure medications should be continued unless changed by your Primary Care Physician. Blood sugar medications can often be decreased very quickly after surgery. Diabetics should continue to monitor your blood sugars and contact your family physician for any questions.
- Initially after surgery you will likely receive pain medications through your IV, but once you are recovering well, this will be switched to pain pills. When you go home, it is ok to "break up" your pain pill if you desire.

Follow-Up Appointment:

If you do not already have a scheduled appointment with your bariatric surgeon, please call his/her office to schedule your postoperative appointment (usually 10-14 days after the date of your surgery).

Pain Control:

Most people who have surgery have some degree of discomfort related to the operation. How much pain you experience has to do with many things: where the incision is, how much manipulation needed to be done in the area, how you usually respond to pain, and how effectively you manage turning, deep-breathing and other activities.

Given that some discomfort is likely, one of our goals is to help you manage the post-operative pain with medication until it begins to go away with healing. A very good thing to remember is that operative pain is LIMITED. After the first few days, you should notice longer and longer periods of less and less pain! People describe surgical pain as burning at the incision site, aching of deeper organs, throbbing or soreness, but only you can describe your pain.

Remember

Whatever method or route of administration is used to manage pain, some general statements are true:

1. Post-operative discomfort is limited. Every day you will notice some improvement. However, after an operation, it is not unusual to have some twinges of pain off and on for several months.

2. It is important to use pain medication as prescribed. That means taking it before pain gets out of control. You will not become addicted. Using pain medicine can actually help you heal faster by allowing you to relax and improve breathing, circulation, appetite and your ability to move around and regain your strength.

3. Plan your activities with pain management in mind. If you know that it takes 20 minutes for your pain medicine to start working, ask for it when you are getting ready to walk, or cough and deep-breathe. You will be better able to manage these activities if your discomfort is under control.

4. Pain medication is designed to manage discomfort; it may or may not eliminate it. It is your job to let us know how the medicine is working so that we can evaluate your progress. Do not assume that we know how you feel. Sometimes we can guess well, but YOU are the only one who can fully evaluate your own comfort.

5. Pain medicine tends to make people constipated. Taking in enough fluids can help. Constipation can make anyone feel terrible! It is generally "ok" to take over the counter medi-

cations for constipation. If you are having problems, let us know.

6. There are many ways of helping reduce your pain that you can actively do yourself. Moving around in bed, walking in the hall, or sitting up in a chair can decrease the aches, pains and weakness that go along with staying in bed. People who are up and around quickly feel better sooner. Watching television, listening to music or tapes, reading, and visiting with friends and family are important ways to increase your comfort level. We all know that taking our mind off things is a great way to deal with discomfort. Use these techniques frequently to help yourself feel better and to make the time pass more quickly! Relaxation techniques such as controlled deep breathing and concentrating to relax specific muscle groups can be helpful. It is not unusual after surgery to subconsciously tense the area of your incision. This can lead to a lot of soreness and aching.

Post-Operative Follow-Up

After surgery, you will be following up with your bariatric surgeon and gradually getting back into your post-operative educational program within a few weeks. This usually includes individualized counseling appointments, behavior modification classes and fitness classes once you are permitted to attend by your bariatric surgeon. Don't forget to take advantage of any post-operative personal training visits that are offered as well. These certified trainers can ease you into fitness so it is non-threatening and enjoyable!

Post-Operative Visits - 10-14 Days

Prior to surgery you will usually be scheduled for your first post-operative visit. Most patients look forward to this visit and your first documented weight after surgery. At this visit, you and your surgeon will discuss your progress on the liquid diet, your bowel/urinary habits, the improvement of your post-operative pain, and your overall health. He/she will check your incision site. If steri-strips are present on your incision, feel free to pick them off as they loosen.

Everyone wants to know how much weight they should lose by this visit. There is no right answer to that question because it varies for everyone. It is dependent upon how much you were overweight prior to surgery, your medications, your gender, and your adherence to the liquid diet/ambulation recommendations. On average, we see a weight loss from 5 -30 pounds at this first visit. We are not as concerned about the "numbers" as much as we are about the percentage of weight you have lost (of your excess body weight) and the progression of your weight loss graph.

Your surgeon will take time to answer any questions you may have and at the end of the visit you will likely be scheduled to come back to the office 2 weeks later (approximately 1 month from surgery).

Post-Operative Visits – 1 Month

At this visit, your surgeon will usually discuss your progress of your puree diet, your bowel/urinary habits, the improvement of your post-operative pain, and your overall health. He/she will take time to answer any questions you may have. You will have continued to lose weight but the amount will not likely be as much as it was at your previous visit. Your body slows down weight loss after the larger amount of weight is lost during the first 2 weeks after surgery. Your body is trying to fight the weight loss but you will continue to lose weight. You will usually be instructed to follow your puree diet for another two weeks. The more activity you can do the better off you will be in the long run.

At one month after surgery, you can generally do anything you are comfortable doing. This needs to be confirmed with your surgeon since opinions and situations vary. As a general rule, you will want to listen to your body. If it hurts to do something, you probably shouldn't be doing it. At the end of your visit, you will likely be scheduled to come back to the office 1 month later (approximately 2 months from surgery).

Post-Operative Visits – 2 Months

At this visit, your surgeon will usually discuss the progress of your diet, your bowel/urinary habits, and your overall health. He/she will check your incision site and drain sites. Your surgeon will take time to answer any questions you may have. Your surgeon will continue to track your weight loss graph and review it with you so you can also be aware of your progress.

Please continue to ask any questions you may have and in between visits, call your surgeon's office if you have questions. At the end of your visit, you will likely be scheduled to come back to the office 2 months later (approximately 4 months from surgery).

Note that the frequency of visits with your surgeon will vary by his/her preference and your particular recovery status. In between these visits you will likely also be meeting with an expert counselor/coach/personal trainer on your surgeon's team.

Brenda Nickel Testimonial
(lost 60 pounds in 6 months & still losing)

Because I was not the "typical" weight loss surgery patient, or at least what I thought was a typical patient, I really did not even consider it an option until another patient said something to me about it when I was in the gym working out. At first, my feelings were hurt and I was angry. I was angry because I knew that she was right...I did need to do something about my weight. Although I worked out about 5 days a week, ran half marathons, completed obstacle courses, and just about any other type of physical challenge you can think of, I was still at least 60 pounds over a healthy weight for my height.

After I got over myself, I attended a seminar and talked with Dr. Clark and the staff at the Center for Weight Loss Success about the gastric sleeve surgery. I wanted to know how much weight I could realistically expect to lose since I was less than 100 pounds overweight. After much thought and careful consideration, I chose to have the surgery.

I went into the surgery with my eyes wide open. I read everything that Dr. Clark and the staff gave me so that I was prepared not only for the surgery but for the journey that was to follow. I attended all of my counseling sessions, listened to all of the webinars and read every page of the materials provided in the Weight

Management University for Weight Loss Surgery™ program. I also attended, and still attend, their Support Group and I continue to maintain an active lifestyle.

I reached my one-year goal in May 2013 and have even lost a few more pounds since. I feel better than I have in over 24 years. Yes, I am still running races and doing all the physically challenging things that I did before, just with more success and an easier recovery. I have even ventured out and tried new things like boxing and long distance biking. The next thing on my horizon is the Iron Girl Sprint Triathlon. I have wanted to do this race for a long time and I am going to do it this year!

I didn't realize what a change I had made until I recently saw my before and after pictures. One of my biggest struggles was that I could make my body do just about anything I wanted but I couldn't lose the weight. Now that the weight is gone, I can do more than I ever imagined. I have 24 years of catching up to do. Every day is a new adventure...century bike rides, triathlons, Stand Up Paddle Board 10Ks...there is always something new to do to test out the new me.

The most important advice I can give you is that everyone's journey is a little different, but every journey should start with a commitment to changing your lifestyle. Weight Loss Surgery is a "tool" that you and you alone are responsible for maintaining. The Center for Weight Loss Success staff is there to help you, but you have to ask for the help when you need it. There is no reason to take the journey alone; they are there to help! You are the keeper of your own life, why not make it a healthy one? Thank you Dr Clark and Staff for all that you did to support me over the last year. You all are amazing!

BEFORE

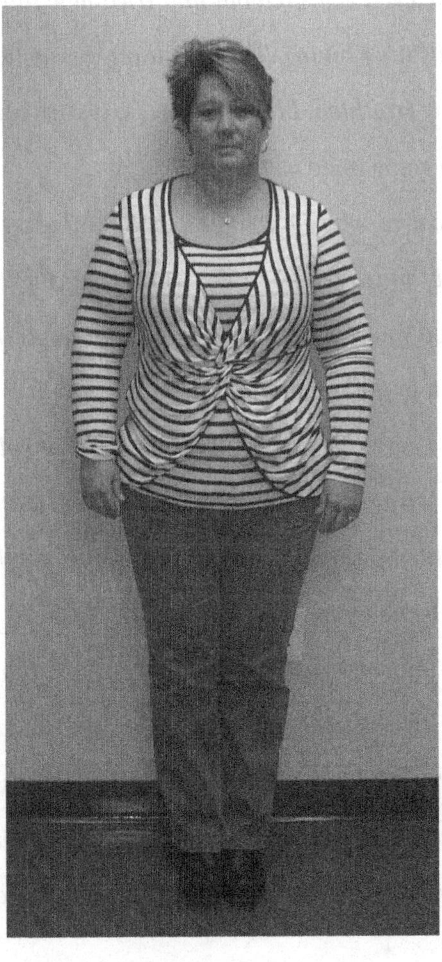

AFTER

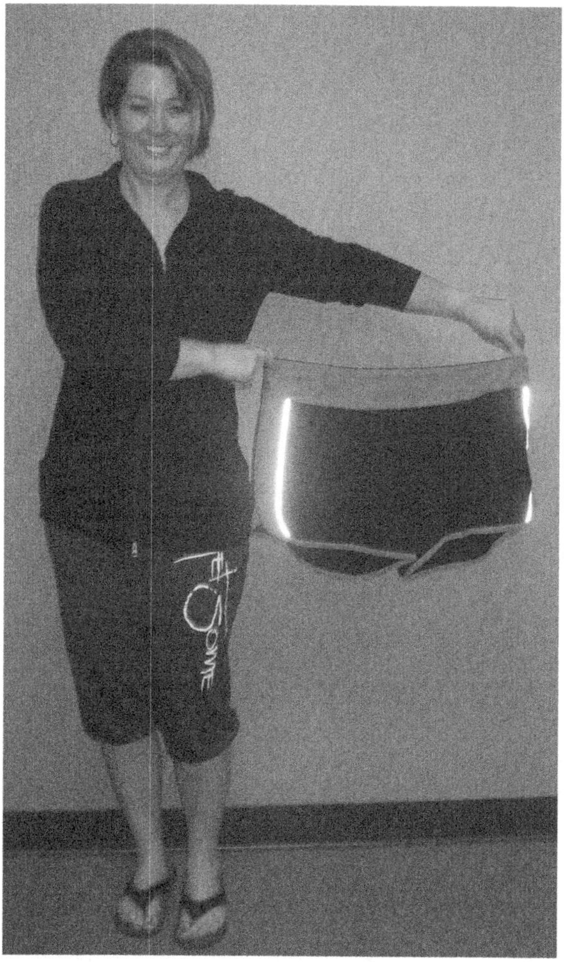

CHAPTER 4

DIETARY GUIDELINES BEFORE SURGERY

Introduction

Please note that this entire chapter includes general guidelines. Your surgeon may or may not recommend a pre-surgery diet and may have a slightly different recommended plan after surgery. You must refer to the orders set forth by your bariatric surgeon and his/her expert team. If you are having surgery at the Center for Weight Loss Success, your ongoing education and Weight Management University for Weight Loss Surgery™ program will be guiding you through this process each step of the way.

The first thing you must realize as you progress toward your surgery date is that this one event, while extremely important, is only just the beginning, and is not an end unto itself. Surgery, as part of a complete weight management program is an effective part of a larger process that will help you in a lifelong commitment to weight loss. With surgery, your health, your weight, your whole well-being will change, but these changes must be understood and, most importantly, be managed by you every day to realize the full potential of the benefits they can bring. The preparation and commitment involved with managing these upcoming changes must occur **before** and **after** the surgery in order to ensure your long-term success.

This chapter outlines a great deal of information regarding why a pre-operative diet is recommended. The evidence is compelling. The chapter also identifies two different meal plans that can be followed for two or more weeks prior to surgery. The first is **Dr. Clark's Jump Start Diet** that utilizes supplements entirely. The second, **Dr. Clark's Quick Fix Plan,** is a 1000-1200 calorie diet which uses food along with some integration of protein supplements (the reason for protein supplementation is explained). Both diets require additional vitamin/nutrient supplements as identified.

Benefits of a Pre-surgery Diet

The main purpose here is to describe what steps **you** can do that will maximize your weight loss and overall health **before** your surgery.

Most people have to wait at least 2-4 weeks (and sometimes longer) from the time they commit to surgery until the actual surgery takes place. This waiting period is an excellent time to undergo a pre-surgery diet. Engaging in a structured weight management plan will benefit you in the following ways:

1. Surgical risk will decrease. The liver and the area around the liver will shrink with initial weight loss. This makes the surgery easier to perform and decreases the risk to you.

2. By modifying your caloric intake before surgery, you will be better prepared for the nutritional lifestyle changes that will occur following your surgery.

3. If you are diabetic, you may be able to reduce, or even stop taking medication before surgery. The same holds true for blood pressure medications.

4. Other conditions associated with obesity, such as chronic back pain, sleep apnea, asthma, and arthritis of the weight bearing joints, will improve with weight loss. The improvement of these conditions before surgery will help your recovery time after surgery.

5. People that make a commitment to lose weight before surgery are generally more committed and therefore more successful after the surgery to attain and maintain their goals for the long-term.

What You Should Know Before You Start the Diet

1. Design of the Diet:

The creation of the pre-surgical diet is the result of years of clinical experience in the weight management field. The final structure of the diet will address not only your nutritional requirements for safe, effective weight loss, but will also take into account your comfort and well-being while on the diet. These last two points are instrumental in your overall success to lose weight, and to maintain that weight loss for the long-term. Essentially, the design of the diet is such that:

- You should not be hungry while on the diet.
- You should have enough energy for work and daily ac tivities while on the diet.
- You should be capable of understanding and following the diet at all times without difficulty.

2. The Role of Protein in the Diet:

The role of protein is **crucial** on a calorie reduced diet.

If you simply go on a reduced calorie diet without adequate amounts of protein, the reduction of your muscle (lean body mass) would be the primary source of weight loss. On reduced calorie diets, your body will draw energy from your lean body mass first, and try to preserve your fat stores as much as possible. Weight loss will be achieved, but a significant portion of your weight loss will be from a depletion of your lean body mass and **not** from your fat stores. In fact, your overall fat **percentage** can actually increase on this type of diet because of the eventual loss of lean body mass, and the retention of fat stores. Besides being ineffective, this type of weight loss will result in a decrease of energy, a decrease in your overall metabolism, and will not work to control your carbohydrate cravings. In addition, if you gain weight back after this type of diet, the weight gain will primarily come back as added fat.

For Example: Suppose that a 5'3" woman weighs 115 pounds, and her percent of fat mass is normal: 25%. Over the next few years, she gradually gains 20 pounds. She now weighs 135 pounds, and her body composition has changed to 35% fat. She goes on a low calorie ("crash") diet and loses 20 pounds in about 6 weeks. Nothing secret about the process – she has basically consumed less than she burns, and she loses weight.

But there is a catch: Her body's natural reaction when protein intake is inadequate is to use her lean body mass as a source of energy to compensate for the calorie depletion, and as a consequence, some of the weight she has lost is muscle. So even though she is back to her original 115 pounds, she is now actually fatter, with a body composition of 30% fat instead of the original 25%.

She then goes back to her "normal" eating habits before her diet and slowly regains the weight she had lost, and is once again at 135 pounds. But the twenty pounds she has regained is not the same pounds she shed, as it is now known that people who regain their weight after "crash" diets usually gain their weight back primarily as fat. Her body composition is now 40% body fat.

If this cycle of losing and regaining weight is repeated several times, her body composition will dramatically change. She will no longer be simply overweight, she will now be over-fat.

To compensate for this, we have designed the pre-surgical diet so that you will receive the required daily amount of protein you need to preserve your lean body mass, as well as a minimum amount of overall calories to maintain energy levels throughout the diet. In addition, the overall daily carbohydrate intake (especially calories from simple carbohydrates) has been sufficiently reduced to promote weight loss and the structure of the menu plans have been designed to help control your carbohydrate cravings. This is particularly important since we find that the majority of our clients suffer from carbohydrate sensitivity (explained on the next page).

Preserving lean body mass through adequate protein intake during the weight loss phase is also the main way to accomplish our two goals of (1) maintaining your energy levels and (2) controlling possible hunger cravings, especially in the later phases, during the entire time weight loss occurs.

Carbohydrate Sensitivity and Its Symptoms

1. Who has carbohydrate sensitivity?

Two thirds of the American population is sensitive to carbohydrates. As weight increases, the percentage of people with a carbohydrate sensitivity condition increases. Consequently, up to about 90% of our surgical patients suffer from carbohydrate sensitivity. It is very common and almost anyone can have it. Carbohydrate sensitivity is also common with diabetics and clients who have a strong family history of diabetes. It is important to note that 95% of Type 2 diabetics are significantly overweight, so obesity has a very important role in carbohydrate sensitivity. It also occurs in women with polycystic ovaries.

2. What are the symptoms of carbohydrate sensitivity?

The symptoms of carbohydrate sensitivity are similar to

hypoglycemia (low blood sugar), and are characterized by the following:

- Cravings
- Hunger
- Fatigue or Sleepiness
- Sweating
- Dizziness
- Headaches

3. What is the cause of these symptoms?

The symptoms are likely directly related to the consumption of refined, simple carbohydrates, especially those carbohydrates consumed without protein in the earlier part of the day.

The pancreas normally secretes insulin in 2 phases – an immediate phase and a delayed phase. People with carbohydrate sensitivity have an absent or blunted initial phase response. The following sequence likely occurs to bring on these symptoms.

- Breakfast of carbohydrate which is primarily lacking in protein, and which is made up of refined, or simple carbohydrates (baked goods, most cereals, fruit)
- Blood sugar rises rapidly to (for example) 160 instead of 120 – because initial phase does not work
- In ½ to 2 hours, pancreas recognizes the 160 blood sugar (elevated, but not in diabetic range) and secretes a large amount of insulin

- Blood sugar **rapidly** falls and produces one or more of the symptoms listed above

In has been shown that it is the **speed of the fall** rather than the amount of the fall that produces these symptoms, and that these symptoms are real and not just in the mind, and something has to be done about them (i.e. eat). The usual case is to eat more of what was just consumed before, and the cycle begins again.

What carbohydrates cause this to happen?

Any food potentially can make this happen, but it is primarily starches (especially refined flour, breads and pastries) and simple sugars that cause the symptoms of carbohydrate sensitivity. The carbohydrate molecules in most starches are a long string of glucose molecules (amylose) that are quickly broken down to glucose and absorbed. Fruits, especially those with high sugar content, are almost as bad. The sugar in them is fructose which is converted in the liver to glucose.

Vegetables are also carbohydrates but they have complex sugars which take time to be digested. High fiber vegetables slow the absorption process down so it takes more volume to get much glucose. Protein can also be converted to sugar in the liver, but this takes more time so the glucose converted from the protein feeds slowly into the blood stream and evens out the blood sugar levels.

4. How are the symptoms of carbohydrate sensitivity avoided?

The diet we are recommending preoperatively allows very little carbohydrate until the evening meal, and then primarily fruits and vegetables. This stops the **swings** in the blood sugar and people with this condition "feel better" almost immediately. Unfortunately, even with the significant weight loss that occurs following surgery, carbohydrate sensitivity does not go away. After weight loss has been completed, carbohydrate sensitivity will still occur, especially if there is any weight regained. Therefore, it is important that you be aware of this condition, and that in addition to watching the overall calories you have eaten, you must realize that the **timing** and **source** of carbohydrates are important for continued weight maintenance.

5. Why is carbohydrate sensitivity so important to recognize?

In weight loss or maintenance, the person without carbohydrate sensitivity only has to learn the number of calories they can eat each day to lose or maintain their weight. If one has carbohydrate sensitivity, he/she will constantly battle hunger during weight loss and maintenance unless he/she (1) avoids carbohydrates (except vegetables) during the first half of the day, or (2) never eats carbohydrate (preferably high fiber carbohydrate) without protein, and also considers (3) eating starches only with the evening meal in very small amounts. This behavior change is very difficult, but extremely important for long-term maintenance.

Terry Steen Testimonial
(lost 85 pounds)

I gained an average of 10 pounds/year once I left the military. After about 7-8 years, I found that I couldn't just diet for a while and get it down like I could in my 20s. After my weight gain slowed, I leveled off about 75 pounds above my comfortable weight. As a result, my health became an issue and my high blood pressure landed me in the hospital for a full week just to get it stable. I started using a low-carb diet and working out to manage my weight and help keep my blood pressure under control. I was on medications, but was making it. A few more years went by and I developed an elevated Hemoglobin A1C, the need for a CPAP machine to sleep, and the beginnings of an enlarged heart.

I had watched my father suffer from these things. I was not able to lower my weight down with methods that used to work so I decided that I was going to do whatever it took to be able to live a normal life again. It took 5 years of thinking about it, but only 2 serious warnings from my doctor to make the commitment to move forward with weight loss surgery.

My insurance required a year of waiting to qualify for surgery. During that year, I had regular meetings with a life coach, diet counseling, joined a support group, and was evaluated mentally and physically. I focused on where I was going to be, what my goals were, and what my new life would be like. I NEVER, NOT ONCE saw surgery as the solution, the fix. I knew it was a tool and I needed to learn how to use that tool to meet my goals.

When I first started investigating weight loss surgery, a web-search or two gave me the names of ALL the bariatric surgeons in the area, state and country. I asked for references from doctors and nurses helped as well as seeing the facility. However, for me, knowing that Dr. Clark approaches weight loss from a whole person perspective and truly a "changing your life" point of view made a huge difference. My personal doctor and I were very pleased with the extensive classes, support groups, and follow up programs he offers (Weight Management University for Weight Loss Surgery™). This made my choice easy.

I have lost 85 pounds over the past 8 months since having weight loss surgery and feel wonderful. Weight loss surgery is not an "easy fix". You need to understand that although you may still want to eat the same foods in the same way, you can learn how to use your new "tool" to control your previous habits. This has been a challenge for me because I have severe carbohydrate sensitivity. This means that I have a tendency to crave when I am not really hungry. I love that I am free of the weight, and so thankful that I now understand how to manage the enemy that tries to make me unhealthy again...that little craving that could push me over the edge. Stay the course! It's very worth it in the end.

BEFORE

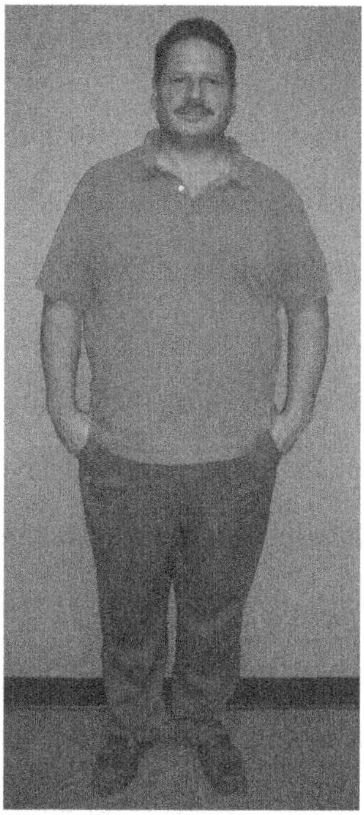

AFTER

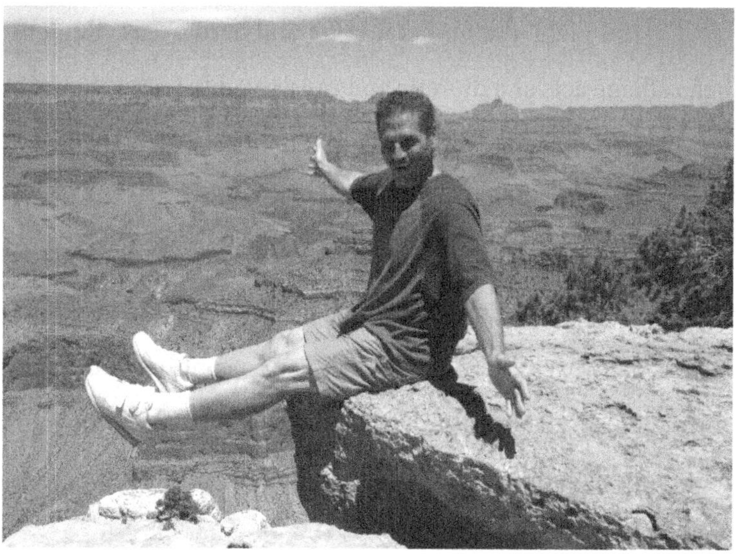

Suggested Vitamins and Other Recommendations

There are certain deficiencies associated with low calorie diets that may bring on unwanted side effects. There are specific dietary supplements that are designed to improve the side effects that may occur during the weight loss phase (i.e. multivitamin, B-complex, Magnesium/Potassium, Essential Fatty Acids, Chromium polynicotinate). Dr. Clark recommends these for anyone in a weight loss program. Your health care team can assist you in determining what supplements are best for you.

You should try to drink ***at least*** 8 cups (64oz) of water each day. You can drink other beverages as long as they are calorie-free (less than 5 calories per serving) and caffeine-free. Suggestions for these types of beverages include decaf coffee and tea, Crystal Light, diet mineral water and herbal teas. Remember, caffeine acts as a diuretic and causes you to lose water from your body. Caffeine also tends to stimulate your appetite. If you must have caffeine, please limit to one serving per day.

At the Center for Weight Loss Success, we recommend that all of our clients **begin journaling** your food and fluid intake as well as daily exercise. We will want you to continue journaling throughout your weight loss journey to help you become more conscious of your food selections and intake - and to track your success!

Protein Requirements and the Use of Supplements

The most important fact that you must realize while you are on the pre-surgery diet is that your daily protein requirements go up. In general, the **minimum** daily protein requirements for a low calorie diet (700-1,200 calories a day) to maintain lean body mass is approximately 90 grams a day for women and 110-120 grams a day for men.

All protein supplements were **NOT** created equal. We encourage you to utilize the products recommended by your surgeon and his/her expert team. Quality supplements are available at the on-site CFWLS nutritional store or online at www.cfwls.com. We use protein based supplements made by companies that specialize in protein supplements made specifically for weight loss.

The protein based supplements will play a crucial role in the structure of your pre-surgery diet by supplying you with the needed protein without adding calories from carbohydrates or unnecessary fat. With the protein supplements, it is extremely simple to calculate and fulfill your daily protein requirements. The servings can be prepared quickly and easily at any location.

Your use of the protein supplements **before** surgery will also help prepare you for your dietary needs **after** surgery. This is especially important during the early stages of your diet just after surgery occurs. You will find that establishing your feeding schedule for your protein requirements (and hydration requirements) will be much easier because of your familiarity of the protein based products.

In addition to the obvious changes in appetite that comes with surgery, you may find that your tolerance levels toward certain foods must be learned all over again. We have found most surgery clients undergo significant changes with respect to their sensory perception. Certain flavors and textures, even smells that were once tolerable can become unpleasant or unbearable after surgery occurs. The protein supplements were specifically developed with the surgery client in mind by creating flavors and textures that are compatible with the changes in taste that frequently occur following surgery. The ease of ingesting protein supplements has further been facilitated by keeping portions as small as possible, with very little or no sugar, while keeping protein levels as high as possible.

Dr. Clark's "Enhanced Jump Start" Diet

1000 Calorie Controlled Carb/Low Calorie Diet

(Using Weight & Inches Meal Replacement Shakes)

This 14 day jump start diet was developed to jumpstart weight loss and decrease the potential risks with undergoing weight loss surgery. One of the most common problems which overweight clients have is fatty liver disease. This can eventually lead to liver failure. The fatty liver is enlarged. This makes the procedure much more difficult to perform which increases risk with the surgery. One of the most important things that you can do **prior** to surgery is to decrease the amount of fat within the liver (which will shrink it in size). This decreases the risk with surgery and jump starts your weight loss program.

The diet uses all supplements to control both the amount of calories and protein. Protein is very important to prevent loss of lean body mass (LBM) during this diet plan. We have also added the appropriate vitamins and minerals which can be continued post-op as well. **Of note – this diet can be used at any time during your weight loss journey to "jump start" your weight loss plan. It can also be continued for longer than 2 weeks if desired since we use true meal replacements.**

Fatigue can occasionally be problematic during aggressive

weight loss plans. Getting protein in and taking vitamins/minerals as prescribed can help avoid this. Adding the combination of a Multivitamin, Essential Fatty Acids (EFA's), Activated B-Complex and Magnesium/Potassium will help prevent fatigue associated with aggressive diet plans.

Weight and Inches (W&I) shakes are made with casein protein which is digested very slowly and subsequently controls hunger quite well. Since the shakes are quite filling, you may divide them up into smaller portions. The shakes come in 2 flavors (chocolate and vanilla). They should be mixed with water (not milk since this adds too much carbohydrate and almost doubles the calories). Adding a tiny amount of other flavor extracts can add some variety to them. Using a blender and ice makes a thicker, frothier/smoother shake and tends to be more filling than just mixing the package with water.

Dr. Clark's "Jump Start" Diet

5 Shakes*/Day (Breakfast, Lunch, Dinner & 2 Snacks)

	Weight & Inches Shake	Calories	Protein (g)	Carbohydrate (g)	Fat (g)
Breakfast	W&I Shake	200	29	15	3
Snack	W&I Shake	200	29	15	3
Lunch	W&I Shake	200	29	15	3
Snack	W&I Shake	200	29	15	3
Dinner	W&I Shake	200	29	15	3
TOTAL		**1000**	**145**	**75**	**15**

To get the most out of this plan, I recommend adding these 3 additional vitamins/nutrients:

- Complete Multi-Vitamin (2 tabs/day)
- Activated B-Complex (1-2 capsules/day)
- Magnesium/Potassium Aspartate (1 twice/day)

Please do not use Essential Fatty Acids (EFA's) for 10 days prior to surgery since they act as a blood thinner. You may also want to consider adding B-Complex injections to help prevent fatigue, commonly associated with calorie restricted diet plans.

Dr. Clark's Quick Fix Plan

This is a food and protein supplementation diet consisting of approximately 1100-1200 calories depending on food choices selected. It is ideal for individuals who wish to "accelerate" their weight loss and get on the right track with a flexible healthy eating plan. The afternoon snack may be taken mid-morning instead. Although, developed as a 2 week "Quik Fix" plan, since it is so nutritionally complete, the plan may be continued longer.

Breakfast (200 calories): 1 Weight and Inches shake

Lunch (200 calories): 1 Weight and Inches shake

Afternoon Snack (200 calories): 1 Weight and Inches shake

If you prefer, you can have one of the CFWLS protein bars for an afternoon snack instead of the third Weight & Inches Shake. However, the bars (though convenient) have more calories and carbohydrates. I recommend using no more than 1 bar per day.

Main Meal (approx. 500-600 calories): Include protein, salad, and vegetable.

Protein (approx.. 250-300 calories): 1 serving daily (approx.. cooked weight) from the following with all skin, bone, visible fat removed and use a cooking method that does not add fat.

- 5 oz ground beef (lean 10%), very lean steak, veal or pork
- 6 oz chicken or turkey (white meat only)
- 6 oz venison or lean ham

- 6-8 oz white fish, shell fish, or canned fish (must be water packed or rinsed)

Salad (approx. 50-100 calories):

- 2 cups lettuce or other leafy greens
- 1 cup vegetables (celery, tomato, cucumber, etc.)

AND

- Low calorie dressing (25 calorie limit) OR vinegar, salt, lemon juice and other desired spices

Vegetables (approx. 50-100 calories):

- Choose 1 cup cooked broccoli, spinach, beets, asparagus, carrots, green beans or cauliflower

Water/Beverages

TRY TO DRINK at least 8 cups (64oz) of water each day.

You can drink other beverages as long as they are calorie-free (less than 5 calories per serving) and caffeine-free. Suggestions for these types of beverages include decaf coffee and tea, decaf diet soda, Crystal Light, diet seltzer or diet mineral water, and herbal teas. Remember, caffeine acts as a diuretic and causes you to lose water from your body. If you must have caffeine please limit to one serving per day.

Journaling

We recommend that all patients begin journaling your food and fluid intake as well as daily exercise using a journal. We will want you to continue journaling throughout your weight loss journey to help you become more conscious of your food selections and intake – and to track your success!

To get the most out of this plan, I recommend these 3 additional vitamins/nutrients that are included in this diet:

- Complete Multi-Vitamin (2 tabs/day)
- Activated B-Complex (1-2 capsules/day)
- Magnesium/Potassium Aspartate (1 twice/day)

Please do not use Essential Fatty Acids (EFA's) for 10 days prior to surgery since they act as a blood thinner. You may also want to consider adding B-Complex injections to help prevent fatigue, commonly associated with calorie restricted diet plans.

Please note: All protein products from the Center for Weight Loss Success have very low sugar in them and all have at least 12-15 grams of protein in them. This makes it possible for them to be interchangeable. Remember to verify the specific nutritional recommendations set forth by your bariatric surgeon.

CHAPTER 5

NUTRITION

Please note that this entire chapter includes general guidelines. You must refer to the orders set forth by your bariatric surgeon and his/her expert team. If you are having surgery at the Center for Weight Loss Success, your ongoing education and Weight Management University for Weight Loss Surgery™ program will be guiding you through this process each step of the way.

The purpose of this section is to show you what foods to eat after surgery to allow your new stomach pouch to heal and guide you in forming new healthy eating habits for life. Contrary to popular belief, nutrition after weight loss surgery is not difficult. It is important that you remember a few key points:

- **Remain hydrated (low calorie/no calorie liquids– Water is BEST!)**
- Work on getting an adequate intake of protein (**at least** 90-100 gms/day)
- Be sure to use your journal every day to track your in take, activity, goals and weight loss
- Sip slowly!
- Follow the progressive diets as outlined in this section (liquid diet for 2 weeks, soft/pureed diet for the next 2-4 weeks, ***low sugar/starch, controlled fat*** diet thereafter)
- When starting real food, cut it up tiny (about the size of a pencil eraser) and chew thoroughly (25-30 chews per bite)
- Don't gulp or overfill your pouch – make sure the cur rent bite is sitting well before you take the next bite

At the end of this chapter, you will have a good understanding of the foods allowed in each stage of your diet (Liquid Diet, Soft/Puree Diet, and Regular Diet) following surgery and the quantity permitted.

You have made an important decision to undergo weight loss surgery. This is an excellent time to "wipe the slate clean" and form new and improved, healthy eating habits for life. In order to have the best possible outcome, special attention must be given to your nutritional status *before and after* surgery. So start now. The healthier you are prior to surgery, the better your chances are for a speedy recovery.

Weight loss surgery provides you with a tool to lose weight. How successful you are depends upon how well you use this tool. You've chosen a path towards better health and wellness – congratulations!

Why is protein important?

Protein is essential for muscle and tissue growth and repair. If you reduce your caloric intake without consuming the necessary amount of protein, your weight loss will be a combination of lean body mass and fat loss. With adequate protein intake (and exercise), you should be able to preserve your muscle mass, allowing the majority of your weight loss to come from fat stores. If, over time, you do not meet your daily protein needs, you may experience fatigue, loss of lean body mass, and possible hair loss.

How much protein do I need?

We recommend that our patients take in **at least 90-100 grams of protein every day.**

As your weight loss continues, your body will still prefer using your lean muscle as a source of energy. Therefore, consuming 90-100 grams of protein daily will be a goal throughout your weight loss journey, not just during the beginning phases.

Once your weight has stabilized and you are in a maintenance phase then protein requirements may decrease somewhat into the 60-90 range depending on your weight and overall muscle mass. The higher your weight the more protein you may require in order to maintain Lean Body Mass. Men typically require more protein due to their higher total Lean Body Mass.

How much should I eat?

Your new stomach pouch will initially only be able to hold about 1-2 tablespoons (15-30cc) of fluid at a time. This is approximately ½-1 medicine cup. Your new stomach should eventually stretch to accommodate 6-8 ounces (3/4 to 1 cup) within the first 1-2 years after surgery. Because your new stomach pouch is so small, you need to follow the guidelines provided to ensure the fluid/food you put in your stomach is the most nutritious possible and does not overfill your small stomach, causing you pain and/or nausea/vomiting.

How often should I eat?

Throughout the *liquid and soft/puree stages* of your new diet, you should sip on low or no calorie liquids **all day long** (water is best). During these stages, you should take in no more than 4 ounces every thirty minutes. When you start "real food" follow eating (but not necessarily drinking) with a thirty minute rest period where you have no intake at all. The rest time allows the food to empty from your small stomach to the small intestines. This decreases the risk of overfilling your stomach as you start drinking liquids again. Over time, as your small stomach expands to accommodate more food, you may eat a little more and have longer rest times so you are no longer eating so frequently, but every 2-3 hours throughout the day. **Eventually (over a number of months), you will be eating three (3) meals a day with a small, planned snack in between meals.**

Low Sugar, Low Fat Liquid Diet

(for use first 14 days after surgery)

Please note that this entire chapter includes general guidelines. You must refer to the orders set forth by your bariatric surgeon and his/her expert team. If you are having surgery at the Center for Weight Loss Success, your ongoing education and Weight Management University for Weight Loss Surgery™ program will be guiding you through this process each step of the way.

This diet is specifically designed for patients who have had weight loss surgery. It will provide you with the energy, protein, and fluid necessary to meet your specific nutritional needs. You will follow this diet for the **first 14 days** after your surgery until I or your surgeon advances your diet at your first post-operative appointment.

General Rules to Follow During This Time:

- **STAY HYDRATED:** During these first few weeks after surgery, we are most concerned that you are hydrated. Try to consume 4-6 cups of fluid per day (remember - your protein drinks count toward your total fluid requirements).
- **DO NOT GULP:** Sip your liquids slowly, taking about 15 minutes to consume 2 ounces. It should take you about one hour to drink 1 cup (8oz) of liquid.

- Transfer your liquids to a one-ounce medicine cup or use a teaspoon to help ensure you sip slowly.
- We do **not** recommend using straws since this often causes you to swallow air along with the liquid which may cause discomfort.
- Do **not** drink carbonated beverages. The carbonation can cause abdominal distension and pressure on your new stomach pouch.
- **TAKE VERY SMALL BITES:** For foods requiring a spoon, use a baby spoon to get in the habit of eating slowly.
- Drink your liquids while sitting up.
- Do **not** lie down right after eating/drinking.
- Stop eating/drinking if you feel full, feel nauseated, or have pain in your shoulder or upper chest.
- Please pay attention to the sugar content in various foods, including the protein supplements. Some are high in sugar, which may cause "dumping syndrome.

Most patients are overwhelmed immediately after surgery. This will get better! As we mentioned before, during these first 1-2 weeks, it is most important to ***stay hydrated.*** Remember to go slowly and do the best you can. You want to get the liquids in and have them stay down. Thus, be careful not to go too fast, take in too much volume, too much fat/sugar or ingest the wrong texture (should be as liquid as possible).

Listed below are protein supplements we have reviewed and consider to be appropriate for use to meet your nutritional needs following weight loss surgery.

Protein Supplements:

Protein supplements are best taken in relatively small doses throughout the day (15-30 gm. at any one sitting). The protein products available through our office are all designed specifically for weight loss and post weight loss surgery. A wide variety can be found in our on-site store or can be purchased online at www.cfwls.com.

SAMPLE MENU – LOW SUGAR, LOW FAT LIQUID DIET

The following are all protein supplements which can be found at our office or the CFWLS e-store. These are only examples. There are multiple protein products that can be used. Please discuss this with the CFWLS store personnel for suggestions and appropriate alternatives.

Breakfast:	1 Cappuccino hot drink mix
Snack:	1 Ready to Drink - Vanilla
Lunch:	1 Cream of tomato soup
Snack:	1 Peach Mango Drink
Dinner:	1 Chicken Broth
Snack:	1 Strawberry pudding/shake

This menu provides approximately 600-700 calories, 90 grams of protein, and 6 cups of fluid. Between supplements, feel free to sip on no calorie beverages or other approved liquids.

Additional Protein Supplements:

If you prefer a different product, we simply ask that you follow a few guidelines. When looking for protein supplements, look for a protein:carbohydrate ratio of at least 2:1 and with low fat. It is also important that you choose a high quality protein, such as whey, soy, casein, or egg protein. If you have specific questions regarding the quality of protein in a particular supplement, **please ask.**

It is important that you remember your protein requirement and drink enough of one or more of the options identified to meet the recommendations. Once you have met your protein needs, you may incorporate other liquids listed on the next page as tolerated.

Low Sugar, Low Fat Liquid Diet

(for use first 14 days after surgery)

Please note that this entire chapter includes general guidelines. You must refer to the orders set forth by your bariatric surgeon and his/her expert team. If you are having surgery at the Center for Weight Loss Success, your ongoing education and Weight Management University for Weight Loss Surgery™ program will be guiding you through this process each step of the way.

FOOD GROUPS	FOODS ALLOWED	FOODS TO AVOID	Comments
MILK/MILK PRODUCTS	Try to avoid use of milk due to the high sugar content (lactose)	All others	8 oz. milk = 8-9 g protein 2 oz. yogurt = 2-3 g protein
VEGETABLES	Tomato juice or "V8 Juice"	All others	4 oz. = 1 g protein
BREAD/ STARCH/ GRAINS	None	All	
FRUITS	100% Juices only (dilute ½ water, ½ juice) Limit use due to high sugar content.	All others	Try to AVOID due to high sugar content
MEATS	None	All	
FATS	None	All	
BEVERAGES	Decaffeinated coffee or tea Sugar free fruit flavored beverages (Kool-Aid, Tang, Crystal Light, etc.)	All others	

DESSERTS	Sugar free flavored gelatin or popsicles Small amounts of sugar free and fat free frozen yogurt or ice milk	All others	Look at labels and determine based upon amount consumed
SEASONINGS	Salt or salt substitute	All others	
SOUPS	Clear broth or Bouillon, Tomato Soup	All others	Look at labels and determine based upon amount consumed
SWEETS	Sugar substitutes or sugar free jelly (no seeds) can be used to top puddings or to flavor plain yogurt	All others	Minimal protein
PROTEIN POWDERS	Any of the protein shakes, drinks, or soups from the CFWLS on-site or online store.	All others	Look at labels and determine based on amount consumed

Soft/Puree Diet

(For use 2-4 weeks after liquid diet)

Please note that this entire chapter includes general guidelines. You must refer to the orders set forth by your bariatric surgeon and his/her expert team. If you are having surgery at the Center for Weight Loss Success, your ongoing education and Weight Management University for Weight Loss Surgery™ program will be guiding you through this process each step of the way.

Gastric Reduction Surgery was developed to induce weight loss. However, you must modify some behavior patterns and eating habits in order to achieve and maintain the desired weight loss in making your operation successful. The gradual re-introduction of food is a carefully staged procedure.

The liquid diet you have been following the past two weeks has helped your new stomach pouch rest and heal. Hopefully you have been able to eat/drink enough fluid and protein each day. It is important that you continue to eat/drink even if you don't feel "hungry". In fact, most patients do not feel true hunger until at least 2-3 months after surgery. Thus, at this point you may not feel hunger, but your body still needs enough calories to support your activity and continue the healing process. Over the next few weeks you may notice that you are able to eat/drink a little more – a good indication that the swelling has gone down from surgery. If **tolerated,** you may now progress to Soft/Pureed foods (the next stage of your diet). **You will usually be instructed to follow this diet for the next 2-4 weeks.**

Pureed food is important for several reasons. After surgery the gastric pouch is swollen, and large portions of poorly chewed food will not pass through the stomach properly. These food particles can block the exit of the pouch and create discomfort. Pureed food prevents the possibility of having large portions of food stick in the stomach. The pureed diet is also helpful for patients who have dentures. Dentures can be a problem in getting food chewed into small particles. These particles could potentially get caught in the pouch.

The diet starts out slowly by using one-ounce medicine cups to portion your food. You may also want to use a baby spoon to get into the habit of eating slowly and not "GULPING" your food. "GULPING" is a common eating problem with Americans, particularly when we eat "on the go". Overcoming "GULPING" will help you learn to eat without experiencing discomfort.

Using the medicine cup will allow you to "eyeball" the amount of food you are taking in so that you can judge how much you should put on your plate when eating regular food a few weeks from now. It is important to remember to eat **slowly** because the eating patterns of your previous years will be too much for your new stomach to handle. Also, because of the small volume of food you will be consuming, you cannot meet all your vitamin needs through food alone. So, you will also need to continue to take your vitamin/mineral supplements as directed.

The most important part of your diet is protein. Below we have listed high protein foods you may try during this stage. Although you will now be getting protein from solid food, most people will need to continue the use of protein supplements at this time in order to consume the recommended 90 grams of protein per day. You may use **finely ground up** scrambled egg, egg salad, tuna salad, chicken salad, refried beans, chili, shredded cheese or cottage cheese.

SAMPLE MENU – SOFT/PUREE DIET

Breakfast:	2 medicine cups (2 oz.) pureed egg or egg substitute
Snack:	1 serving protein drink/shake
Lunch:	2 medicine cups (2 oz.) fat-free refried beans
Snack:	4 oz. low fat, low sugar yogurt
Dinner:	2 medicine cups (2 oz.) pureed tuna with 2 tsp. light mayo
Snack:	1 protein supplement drink/shake

This menu provides approx. 750 calories and over 90 grams of protein. Between meals, you will need sip on an additional 4-6 cups of fluid, for a total of 6-8 cups of fluid a day.

Any other food that is desired after protein needs are met can consist of **pureed vegetables or pureed fruits.** Fruits should be kept to a minimum due to the high sugar content which will slow weight loss. Most patients can eat 1½ to 3 medicine cups of pureed products with each meal. Keep your foods low sugar.

Throughout the soft/puree stage of your diet you should drink or eat no more than 4 ounces in a thirty minute period (i.e. go slow). Follow eating (but not necessarily drinking) with a thirty minute rest period where you have no intake at all. As your pouch expands to accommodate more food, you may eat a little more and have longer rest times so you are no longer eating frequently, but every 2-3 hours throughout the day.

You should drink 6 to 8 cups (48-64 oz.) of liquid per day IN BETWEEN MEALS. Liquids are needed to replace normal body losses and thus prevent dehydration. These should be no calorie (or very low calorie) liquids. Recommended beverages are **water, tea, coffee and diet NON-carbonated beverages such as sugar free Kool-Aid and Crystal light. Remember, liquid protein supplements also count toward your total fluid needs.**

EAT SLOWLY! The following are hints to help you eat more slowly:

- Set aside at least 30-45 minutes to eat each meal.
- Make an "EAT SLOWLY" sign and place it on the table in front of you.
- If possible, sit near a clock or use a watch to time yourself.

Two to three ounces of pureed food should be eaten in a 20-30 minute period.

• Liquids should not be taken 15 minutes before meals and not until 30-45 minutes after meals. (There is not enough room in your stomach for **both** food and liquids.)

• Explain to family members why you must eat slowly so they will not urge you to eat faster.

• Take very small bites of food. Try eating with a baby spoon.

• Put your eating utensil down in between bites. Pay attention to taste. Learn to savor each bite, noticing its flavor, texture, and consistency.

STOP EATING AS SOON AS YOU ARE FULL! Besides causing you to vomit, extra food over a period of time may stretch your stomach.

INDICATIONS of fullness may be:

- A feeling of pressure or fullness in the center of your lower chest or just below the rib cage.
- Feeling of nausea
- Pain in your shoulder area or upper chest
- Hiccups

If you start vomiting and it continues throughout the day, stop eating foods and just sip clear liquids (sugar free gelatin, sugar free juice with no pulp, broth, coffee, tea, or sugar free

Popsicle.) The vomiting may indicate that your outlet is irritated. If intermittent vomiting continues for more than 24hrs, contact your physician. Most vomiting episodes can be prevented.

THE CAUSES OF VOMITING ARE:

- Eating too fast and not chewing food properly
- A bite that is too big
- Eating too much at a meal
- Drinking liquids right after eating
- Lying down after a meal
- Eating foods that don't agree with you.

IN SUMMARY ... REMEMBER IT IS IMPORTANT TO:

- EAT SLOWLY
- EAT PROTEIN FIRST TO MEET YOUR GOAL
- STOP EATING WHEN YOU ARE FULL
- SIP LOW CALORIE BEVERAGES IN BETWEEN MEALS - Water is best!
- DON'T FORGET TO JOURNAL EACH DAY
- EXERCISE REGULARLY (i.e. walking during the first two weeks after surgery)

The next table lists more specifics regarding recommended food groups for your soft/puree diet. Be sure to review the foods to avoid.

Please note that this entire chapter includes general guidelines. You must refer to the orders set forth by your bariatric surgeon and his/her expert team. If you are having surgery at the Center for Weight Loss Success, your ongoing education and Weight Management University for Weight Loss Surgery™ program will be guiding you through this process each step of the way.

Soft/Puree Diet

(for use 2-4 weeks after liquid diet)

FOOD GROUP	FOOD ALLOWED	FOOD LIMITED	FOODS TO AVOID
MEATS	Pureed tuna, chicken, turkey, veal, pork, beef, lamb, and fish. Shredded low fat cheese (Alpine Lace Mozzarella, "Kraft Free"), puree beans or fat-free refried beans. Use in place of 1oz meat: Soft, cooked or poached egg; soft scrambled egg or egg beaters (1/4 c) cottage cheese (1/4 c) mashed or pureed tofu (3oz).		Commercial baby meat unless they are low in fat.
MILK/MILK PRODUCTS	Sugar free, low fat yogurt (no seeds, pulp or chunks). Sugar free pudding.	Take in between meals at least 30-45 minutes before or after meals. Sip slowly: 2oz in 15 minutes.	All others including milkshakes, malts and eggnog. Keep milk to a minimum due to high sugar content (lactose).

FRUITS	Puree only, all without sugar, seeds, cores, and skins. **Use in very limited amounts.**	Use only after meeting protein needs.	All others
VEGETABLES	Puree only. Frozen mashed squash or canned pumpkin can be used.	Use only after meeting protein needs.	Try to avoid high starch vegetables such as potatoes, peas and corn.
BREADS & STARCHES	None		All
FATS	May use *small amounts* of mayonnaise olive oil, diet spreads, butter and cream.		All others
BEVERAGES	Regular or decaf coffee or tea, sugar free fruit flavored beverages (Kool-Aid, Crystal Light etc…).	Take in between meals 30-40 minutes before or after meals. SIP slowly: 2 oz. in 15 minutes	All others
DESSERTS	Sugar free gelatin/popsicle, sm. amts. fat free, sugar free frozen yogurt or ice milk	Treat these as liquids	All others
SOUP	Clear broth, bouillon, consommés, low fat cream soup	Treat these as liquids	All others
SWEETS	Sugar substitute, sugar free jelly (no seeds) – can use to top puddings or to flavor plain yogurt		All others

The Progression Diet

The soft/puree diet you have been following for the past 2-4 weeks has continued to help your new stomach pouch rest and heal. Keeping your food record should help to make sure you eat/drink enough protein and fluid each day.

You are now ready to try soft cooked foods that are not pureed. You should cut your food up to about the size of a pencil eraser. Continue to eat/drink slowly since your stomach pouch may still only be able to hold very small amounts at a time. It is important for you to closely observe and document your reactions to various foods. These soft cooked foods are no longer pureed and special attention must be given to chewing food thoroughly before swallowing (goal = chew 30 times with each bite). Ground or very soft foods may be necessary if you have dentures or missing teeth.

After you are on this diet for a couple of weeks, you can begin to experiment more with various foods. Introduce raw fruits and vegetables cautiously. Certain foods may be difficult to tolerate because your digestive system cannot handle them. The following may cause problems for you and generally should be AVOIDED:

- Tough meats, especially hamburger. Even after grinding, the gristle in hamburger is hard to digest.
- Membranes of oranges or grapefruit

- Cores, seeds, or skins of fruits or vegetables
- Fibrous vegetables such as corn, celery or sweet potatoes
- Hulls, popcorn
- Breads. Fresh breads "ball up" in your stomach and can block your pouch. Try to avoid breads/crackers/cereals as much as possible.
- Fried foods
- Milk – If you are lactose intolerant you may use "Lactaid" products or soybean milk
- Rice
- Breast of Chicken (due to reduced moisture)

REMEMBER TO CONTINUE TO:

1. EAT SLOWLY
2. CUT THINGS UP INTO SMALL PIECES AND CHEW FOOD WELL
3. STOP EATING WHEN YOU ARE FULL
4. "SIP" LOW CALORIE BEVERAGES BETWEEN MEALS
5. SELECT A BALANCED DIET
6. EXERCISE REGULARLY

For successful weight loss after weight loss surgery, changes in **YOUR** eating habits are a must. The operation alone is not a cure. You will **not** be able to lose as much weight as you would like if you eat continuously (grazing), or if you stretch your stomach by eating large amounts of food at one time. You will achieve **YOUR** desired weight loss only if **YOU** are willing to control what you eat and the way in which you eat.

SAMPLE MENU - PROGRESSION DIET

Breakfast	1 Serving Weight & Inches or Lean-N-Complete Meal Replacement Shake mixed with water or blended with ice.
Snack	1oz. low fat cheese
Lunch	2 oz. chicken breast, with 2 tsp. light mayo 1 oz. well-cooked vegetable
Snack	1 protein supplement cold drink or protein bar*
Dinner	2 oz. Salmon 2 oz./ chopped, well-cooked vegetable, with 1 tsp. olive oil
Snack	1 protein supplement pudding or protein bar*

This menu provides approximately 850 calories and over 100 grams of protein

*Remember to limit bars to no more than one/day and preferable no more than 5/week.

Progression Diet

FOOD GROUPS	**FOOD ALLOWED**	**FOOD LIMITED**	**FOODS TO AVOID**
VEGETABLES	Well cooked vegetables		Be careful with raw vegetables
BREAD/CEREAL STARCH	Protein based oatmeal or smooth oatmeal with added protein powder.	**Use only after meeting protein needs and preferably whole grains.**	Avoid **ALL** refined carbohydrates such as white bread, rolls & cereal.
FRUIT	Unsweetened and diluted canned or soft fruits and fruit juices in limited amounts!	Limit to 1 portion only per day.	Avoid sweetened canned fruit and fruit juices, pineapple, raisins, figs, and berries
MEAT	TENDER, well cooked meat, poultry or seafood; soft scrambled egg or egg substitute, cottage cheese, low fat cheeses, tofu, soft cooked or poached eggs, beans and lentils		All others
FAT	Butter, margarine, diet spreads, small amounts of mayonnaise, cream cheese, olive oil, non-stick cooking sprays	Limit regular fat to 3 tsp. per day	Avoid fried foods, bacon drippings, greasy gravies, cream sauces

BEVERAGES *Water is best!*	Coffee, unsweetened (or artificially sweetened) tea, sugar free non-carbonated beverages such as Crystal Light	Sip slowly in between meals.	All others
DESSERTS	Small amts. sugar free, fat free ice milk, low calorie custard, yogurt, puddings, sugar free gelatin, sugar free Popsicle		All others
SWEETS	Diet jelly (no seeds), diet syrup, sugar substitute		Avoid jam, jelly, honey, sugar candy
SEASONINGS & MISCELLANEOUS	Salt, ketchup, mustard, vinegar	Use pepper, spices & herbs cautiously	Avoid popcorn

Vitamin/Mineral Supplementation

Multivitamins: Taking vitamins will be a lifelong commitment for all patients who have had weight loss surgery. In the beginning, you should take **two chewable complete multivitamins** each day. At one month after surgery, you may be able to progress to taking two regular vitamins daily. We recommend two vitamins each day during the first year when your weight loss is most rapid. After the first year, you should continue to take one multivitamin a day. Women may want to consider a prenatal vitamin if pre-menopausal.

B-Complex: Usually around 1 month after surgery, we recommend that you also add one B-Complex vitamin each day (or even 2 per day). The B vitamins assist in muscle and nerve functioning and have been shown to increase a person's energy level over time. You cannot overdose on B vitamins. If you take in more than you need, you will simply rid yourself of any excess through your urine. It is common for B vitamins to cause your urine to be darker or a brighter yellow. This is normal. If you prefer, B-Complex is also available as an injection at the office as appropriate.

Essential Fatty Acids (EFA's): Take them – they're just good for you. By taking fish oil supplements, Omega-3 fatty acids are ingested in their biologically active form. They can be directly used to support cardiovascular, brain, nervous system, and immune function. The mini-soft gels are smaller and have a natural lemon flavor to prevent a "fishy" after taste. Our product is ultra-filtered to guarantee removal of mercury and other possible contaminants. Most people should take 2-4 soft gels per day. They are also helpful to prevent constipation.

Magnesium-Potassium: During weight loss your body will tend to waste both magnesium and potassium. Both of these minerals are essential to normal muscular and cardiovascular function. Magnesium is involved in over 300 biological reactions throughout the body. It can help prevent/treat fatigue. If you are prone to muscle cramps – you need to add this supplement. Typical doses are 1-4 tablets daily with food.

Eating Goal

Try to work up to a **1000 calories/day** consumption to provide adequate fuel for your body. Initially you will only consume about 600-800 calories, contributing to approximately ½-1 pound/day weight loss for the first month. As your stomach pouch is able to tolerate more food and your consumption increases, the expected rate of weight

loss is 2-3 pounds/week (second and third month). This will eventually change to 1-2 pounds of weight loss/week (a healthy rate of weight loss).

"Dumping Syndrome"

This term pertains to **gastric bypass clients only,** but all weight loss clients need to avoid sugar. Sugar is found naturally in grains, fruits, vegetables and milk products. This sugar generally will not cause dumping syndrome (defined below). However, added table sugar is not usually tolerated after gastric bypass surgery. Avoid foods and beverages with more than 8 grams of sugar (5 grams if you are Diabetic) per serving.

Dumping syndrome occurs when there is a rapid passage of food into the small intestines causing a shift of fluid to the small intestine. This usually occurs when you ingest foods that are too high in sugar or fat. Symptoms include diarrhea, sweating, nausea, cold/clammy skin, dizziness, weakness, flushed appearance, and occasionally headaches. You will need to stop and rest until the symptoms subside. Remember to remain hydrated (water is best). Take note of the food/foods that caused these symptoms so that you can avoid them in the future.

Alcohol

Alcohol is full of empty calories, dehydrates the body, and has negative effects on the kidneys and liver. In addition, because of the small size of your new pouch and the fact that food/liquid now empties more rapidly into the intestines, alcohol will be more toxic and cause a higher blood alcohol level than before surgery. For these reasons, ingestion of alcohol should be avoided after surgery. If you choose to ingest alcohol, please be aware that a small amount can affect you to a MUCH greater degree than prior to surgery.

Pre-operative Shopping List

Many clients at the Center for Weight Loss Success have requested a "shopping list" for dietary items that will be helpful for the immediate post-surgery liquid diet. It is helpful to purchase items you will utilize when you return home from the hospital so that you do not need to worry about sending someone to the store at the last minute. The items listed below are only suggestions. You do not need to buy everything. This is true especially if you find you do not like the taste of them or if you do not tolerate them well. Purchase items that you feel will work for you. Remember, protein is extremely important over time. However, during the first 14 days after surgery, we are most concerned that you REMAIN HYDRATED and try to get in 90-100 grams of protein per day.

Pre-Operative Shopping List

ITEM	LOCATION
1. Protein Based supplements	Weight Loss Nutritionals On-Site Store
2. Lean-N-Complete meal replacement shakes	Weight Loss Nutritionals On-Site Store
3. Any Whey non flavored whey protein that can be added to other foods	Weight Loss Nutritionals On-Site Store
4. Small Medicine Cups	Sam's Club, Drug Store
5. Chewable Complete Multivitamin	Weight Loss Nutritionals On-Site Store
6. Baby Spoon/Fork	Grocery or Drug Store
7. Low-fat Yogurt (no added sugar, no seeds or chunks of fruit)	Grocery Store
8. Pudding (sugar free)	Grocery Store
9. Sugar Free Kool-Aid, Tang, Crystal	Grocery Store
Light	Grocery Store
10. Sugar Free Jell-O	Grocery Store
11. Sugar Free Popsicles	Grocery Store or Weight Loss Nutritionals
12. Soups – tomato, clear broth	On-Site Store
13. Sugar Substitute	Grocery Store

Jeanette Castaneda Testimonial
(lost 150 pounds)

I have always believed that your children know your deepest thoughts. My oldest son knew the depression that I was dealing with because of my obesity. So, at his encouragement, I decided to look into weight loss surgery. He wanted his mom to be here and healthier for the family that he and his wife were planning to start.

In September, 2011, I attended a seminar with Dr. Clark. I decided to have the gastric sleeve procedure. I weighed 300 pounds. Dr. Clark advised me to lose as much weight as possible before surgery. The procedure was scheduled for Dec. 12th. On the morning of surgery, I weight 275 pounds. Recovery from surgery was a breeze. I followed Dr. Clark's instructions and participated in the comprehensive educational program at his center.

As a part of this, every month I attended counseling with his experienced staff along with my scheduled follow-up visits with Dr. Clark. Each month a new chapter was added to my Weight Management University for Weight Loss Surgery™ notebook which helped me each step of the way as well. Before I knew it, my year was completed!

Today, I am happy to say that I have more than achieved my goal. I weigh 150 pounds. I never thought I would see that day. I went from a size 3X to a size 12 - a medium! I have gained confidence in ME and I am no longer depressed.

Last Mother's Day, I took a motorcycle ride for the 1st time in 35 years. This summer I rode on every single roller coaster at Busch Gardens. I also took my first airplane trip. Of all my goals achieved, the one thing I look forward to most of all now is the arrival of my first grandchild. I am overwhelmed with joy because finally I feel ALIVE, and looking forward to living the new me. Thanks Dr. Clark and all his caring staff!

BEFORE

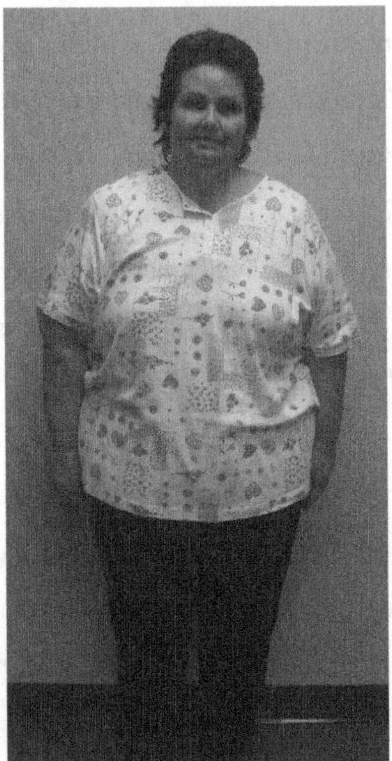

AFTER

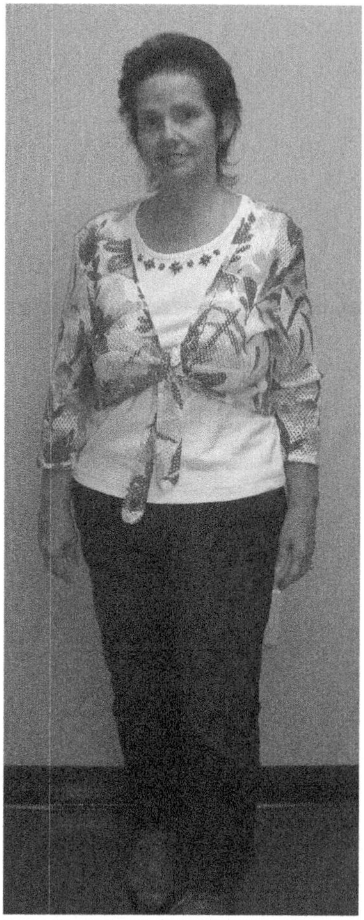

CHAPTER 6

Exercise

Even though you may HATE exercise, please be sure to read this chapter. Exercise is extremely important following weight loss surgery because you will be losing weight at a rapid pace. Your body will try to fight this weight loss by attempting to store fat for this perceived starvation. Your body does this by burning muscle mass and storing fat. This is undesirable. To combat this effect, it is important to **exercise regularly** so that your metabolism is increased and your body burns fat rather than muscle mass.

Now that you have decided to have weight loss surgery,

you should seize this opportunity and integrate activity/exercise into your daily routine. This will not only help you through any plateaus, it will help you build muscle, enhance your metabolism and overall energy, and greatly influence your overall success. You will succeed if you follow many of the guidelines presented in this book. ***Be sure to eat protein first at any meal, drink plenty of water, exercise regularly, and avoid high calorie liquids and "grazing" (snacking) throughout the day.***

We encourage walking beginning the day of surgery to improve circulation. Early walking forces the heart to pump blood throughout the body and prevents it from pooling in your legs which could cause clots that are potentially life threatening. The more walking you can do, the better. We ask that you avoid lifting heavy weights or doing sit-ups/abdominal crunches until you are at least 4 weeks from your surgery. Prior to that time, you may ride an exercise bike, or swim (not until 2 weeks from your surgery). When you choose your particular exercise program, make sure it incorporates weight training along with some form of aerobic/cardiovascular exercise.

Benefits of Exercise (once you are released to exercise by your bariatric surgeon)

Most everyone knows the benefits of exercise – it's just doing it that is difficult. We all can find excuses (not enough time, not enjoyable/boring, inconvenient, lack of resources, don't know how, etc...). The bottom line is that we all must make time for exercise and make it a priority. This is easy to say, but hard to do.

The benefits of exercise are many. Some of these benefits include:

- Decreased appetite
- Decreased blood pressure
- Decreased stress level
- Reduced risk for development of heart disease
- Reduced risk for colon and other cancers
- Reduced depression and anxiety
- Improved balance and independent living
- Improved digestion
- Improved self-esteem
- Improved flexibility
- Improved energy levels
- Improved sleep pattern
- Improved sexual satisfaction
- Improved overall quality of life

So you may logically understand the benefits of exercise. If you still choose not to exercise, you must ask yourself "why?" Determine your roadblocks to exercise and then identify solutions to the roadblock. Once you "get the fever" for exercise after doing some form on a regular basis, you will wonder why you didn't do it earlier. You are making a life changing decision for weight loss surgery. **Now maximize the benefits of this decision and commit to a regular exercise program. You will not regret it and your weight loss will be enhanced and your overall quality of life improved.**

Easing into Exercise

The important thing to remember is that exercise is one of the best things you can do for your health and it is *not acceptable to exclude some form of exercise* during your weight loss process.

It does take time and effort to get started. In addition, you have had surgery which contributes to feelings of fatigue for the first one to three months after surgery. Until you can begin a more vigorous exercise program (4 weeks after surgery), walk as much as possible. If you are unable to walk due to a health problem/disability, perform as much upper body exercise as you can tolerate using light weights (until 4 weeks after surgery). If you have cardiac/respiratory problems, be sure to obtain clearance for starting an exercise program from your primary care physician and/or specialist.

Choose a fitness program that will work for you. It should

be tailored to your specific needs, abilities, preferences and activities that you will enjoy. Otherwise, you will be tempted to quit.

Remember that at the Center for Weight Loss Success, we love making fitness fun and specialize in starting wherever you are. We work privately with you and offer three personal training sessions as a part of your Weight Management University for Weight Loss Surgery™ program. Our certified trainers love working with clients at all levels of fitness. You can also participate in our Group Fitness classes as a part of your program. You are not alone. Please use these resources to enhance your weight loss and improve your overall health and metabolism.

When starting a workout program, take it easy. Be sure to gradually work up to at least 30 minutes of vigorous exercise three or more times a week. Stick to it and strive to make exercise a habit (usually considered a habit once performed regularly for at least three months)! You won't see dramatic changes overnight but you will see dramatic changes over time.

When you exercise, be sure to warm-up prior to the activity and cool down/stretch after the activity. Do not lift too much weight (increase weight gradually), and remain hydrated – be sure to drink water before and after your workout.

Motivation

No one can motivate you except for yourself. You will likely be most successful if you:

- Make a specific plan that fits you and your lifestyle
- Establish a time and place to exercise
- Determine realistic goals (increase your routine gradu ally)
- Choose the right equipment
- Find a partner/buddy to exercise with
- Keep an exercise log
- Reward yourself with something other than food

You can do it!! We say this throughout this book but it is true. You have made a decision to change your life forever in order to attain your particular health goals. Make the most of this first year after surgery and every year thereafter – **you are worth it!**

Kevin Lyles Testimonial

(lost 104 pounds)

From Fatboy to 'Atta Boy' ... I am very happy with the results of my surgery. I've clearly lost more than my mustache and regained my health.

At my heaviest 330 pounds, I might have been a well-dressed big man, but i was often uncomfortable with my belly hanging over my belt and not being able to sit comfortably in a restaurant or airport seat.

I prepared for weight loss surgery and lost 25 pounds before I even went in for the procedure, so I was only 305 pounds. Only ... although I am able to joke about it now at the time it was anything but funny. My blood sugar was never at the right level and I took multiple drugs which were supposed to keep my diabetes, blood pressure and cholesterol levels balanced.

I can hardly believe it even a year out, no insulin since 4 days after the surgery, Type II Diabetes completely under control. Other medications cut in half. Cholesterol down and blood pressure at acceptable levels. The changes are ongoing. Having weight loss surgery not only gained me a healthy lifestyle it changed my social and activity lifestyle as well.

Having the surgery has allowed me to move forward with my martial arts training. I have been taking several different dis-

ciplines for about 6 years now. In addition to no more back pain or knee pain, increased endurance, and greater maneuverability, losing 75 pounds has allowed me to complete requirements for my black belt in Shito-ryu Karate. I take Kendo as well and for the first time my armor actually fits me. I now look forward to the 3 times a week classes and am even helping teach beginning students.

Now I am able to keep up physically. I have increased stamina. I can shop in the regular part of the clothing store where more choices are offered. I look better in my clothes and feel better physically and emotionally. And best of all, I have no more concern about the image I present to business associates, family, my wife's friends or my kid's friends.

As an added benefit, my wife took the opportunity to start eating healthy and working out. She's down about 35 pounds in the last year as well and looks great. With me at 226 pounds, we are actively doing things together to continue to maintain a healthy, happy and energetic life. The hardest part is getting used to the compliments and well wishes.

Surgery was one of the best things I ever did -- for myself, my wife and our two sons.

BEFORE

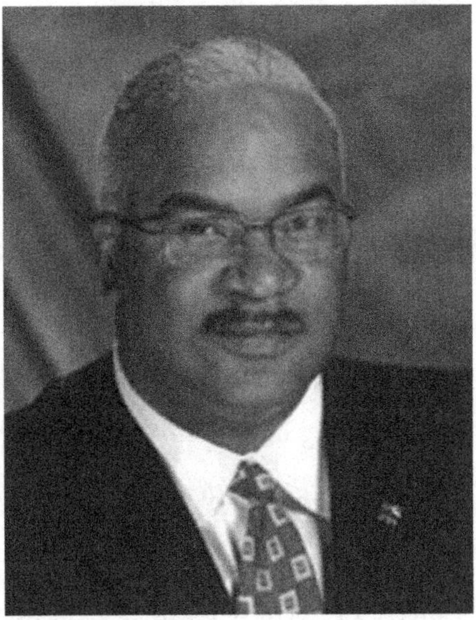

AFTER

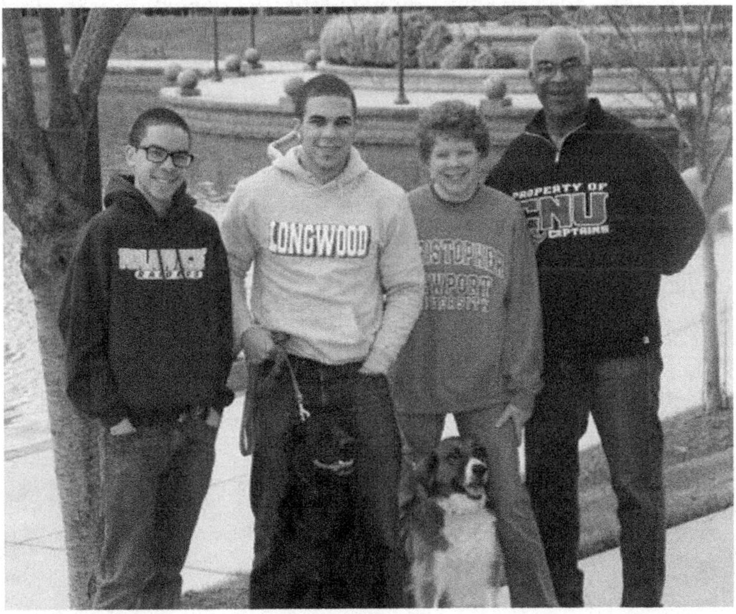

CHAPTER 7

Weight Loss Surgery Procedures

Weight loss surgery is a personal decision and one that hopefully you have investigated and discussed thoroughly with your surgeon. This overview includes the three primary surgical procedures performed within the United States as of the publication of this book along with the advantages, risks and typical results and outcomes for each. These three procedures are the Sleeve Gastrectomy (also referred to as the Gastric Sleeve), the Laparoscopic Adjustable Gastric Banding (also referred to as LapBand® or Realize Band®) and the Laparoscopic Gastric Bypass.

Sleeve Gastrectomy:

The Sleeve Gastrectomy is a newer laparoscopic weight loss surgical procedure in which a small "sleeve-shaped" stomach is created. Approximately 75% of the "stretchy" portion of the stomach is removed. This also removes the portion of the stomach that makes the hormone ghrelin. Ghrelin is a hormone which makes you feel hungry. The remaining "sleeve" of the stomach is about the size and shape of a medium banana. Because anatomy remains normal, this procedure can be considered for people with less weight to lose (50-60 pounds overweight).

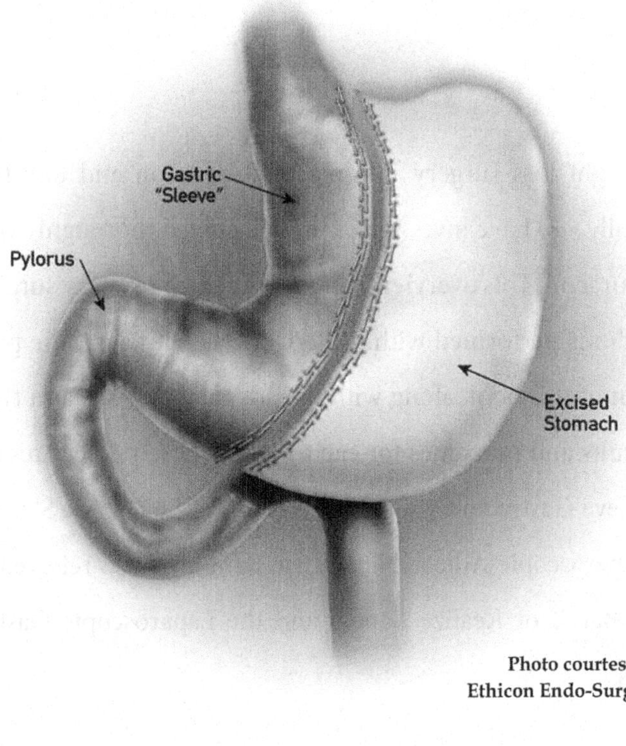

Photo courtesy of Ethicon Endo-Surgery Inc.

Advantages:

- The portion of the stomach that produces ghrelin (a hormone that stimulates hunger) is removed.
- The stomach is reduced in volume, but otherwise tends to function normally.
- **No** "Dumping Syndrome" since the pylorus is pre served.
- **No** intestine is bypassed so there is little chance of nutritional deficiencies.
- **No** implanted device that requires adjusting.
- Procedure is performed laparoscopically most of the time.
- Usually done as an outpatient.

This procedure tends to work due to two major reasons:

1. You have a much smaller stomach and will feel full with eating only a small amount.
2. There is a decrease in the hormone ghrelin so that hunger is controlled much easier.

The sleeve gastrectomy was originally developed as the 1st stage of a 2 stage procedure (patients would undergo a conversion of the sleeve gastrectomy to a bypass procedure). However, it was found to work so well on its own that most patients did not need (or want) to go through with the next stage. This surgery **cannot** be reversed **(i.e. once that part of the stomach is gone…it's gone).**

Risks:

Obesity, age, and other diseases increase your risks from any surgery. Below are identified risks related to surgery and the sleeve gastrectomy procedure based upon national averages:

- Risk of death is 1:500-1,000
- Leaks (1-2%)
- Infection (2%)
- Blood Clot/Pulmonary Embolus (1%)
- Nausea/vomiting
- Peptic ulcer disease
- Formation of gallstones due to rapid weight loss
- Stricture (1%)

Some of these problems may require further surgical intervention.

Typical Results and Outcomes:

Weight loss outcomes are tracked closely at the Center for Weight Loss Success. We are proud that outcomes here generally out-perform national averages. The average best weight loss for this procedure is 65-70% of a client's excess body weight (i.e. if someone is 100 pounds. over their ideal body weight, average weight loss outcomes would be 65-70 pounds).

A weight loss of only about 40% of excess body weight will often show significant improvement in many other medical problems:

- Many Type 2 diabetics will get off of their medications
- Hypertensive clients will have improvement or resolution of their hypertension
- Sleep apnea almost always improves
- Cholesterol improvement in most clients
- Arthritic symptoms improve

Laparoscopic Adjustable Gastric Banding (Lap-Band® or Realize Band®):

The FDA approved adjustable gastric banding surgery in June, 2001. However, it was developed in the 1980's and has been used in Europe since 1993. In terms of surgical procedures for weight loss, this is the least invasive procedure.

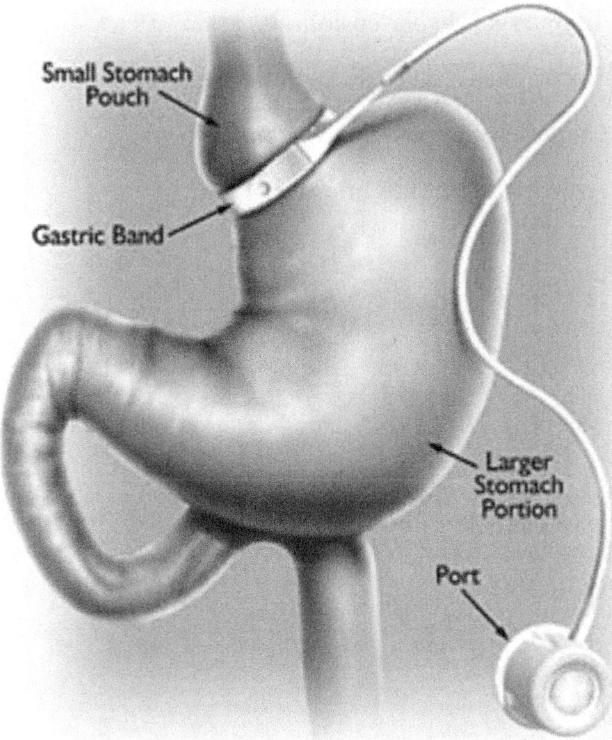

Photo courtesy of Allergan

Laparoscopic adjustable gastric banding involves applying a band around the upper part of the stomach. As a result, this creates a small gastric pouch at the top of the stomach, with a small opening to the rest of the stomach. The band is made of an inflatable silastic ring that controls the flow of food from the small pouch to the rest of your digestive system. With this surgery, there is no cutting or stapling required for dividing the stomach.

In addition to the band, a small port is connected by tubing to the inflatable ring around the stomach. The port is secured just beneath the skin where fluid can be injected or withdrawn to inflate or deflate (adjust) the band. This results in increasing or decreasing the size of the opening between the upper small gastric pouch and the lower portion of the stomach. The need for an adjustment is determined by the surgeon based upon weight loss and symptoms related to eating.

Like any tool, it can be used correctly or incorrectly. Used incorrectly (such as drinking high calorie liquids) you will have relatively poor weight loss or even weight gain. It is still diet, exercise, and behavior change which produce weight loss. Thus, following your surgeon's recommendations are crucial to your overall success.

Advantages:

- Risk of death is approximately 1:1000
- There is no division or re-routing of intestinal tract

- Minimal risk of malnutrition
- The procedure is considered reversible since the Band can be removed with minimally invasive technique if needed

The band is adjustable:

- Often performed under fluoroscopic guidance
- May require 4-6 adjustments during the first year (or more)
- Adjustments need to be checked yearly – **forever**

The band is effective with the following considerations:

- Weight loss success is directly related to:
  - close clinical follow-up
  - appropriate adjustments
  - exercise
  - diet and behavior modification

The potential **<u>disadvantages</u>** of laparoscopic adjustable gastric banding are as follows:

- Weight loss is typically slower when compared to other weight loss surgeries
- Adjustments are required throughout your lifetime
- Problems can develop secondary to the mechanical device

Risks:

Obesity, age, and other diseases increase your risks from any surgery. Below are identified risks related to surgery and the laparoscopic adjustable gastric banding procedure based upon national averages.

- Risk of death is 1:1000
- Infection (<1%)
- Blood Clot/Pulmonary Embolus (1%)
- Gastric pouch dilation potentially requiring further surgery (5%)
- Band slippage or migration often requiring further surgery (5%)
- Band erosion requiring further surgery for band removal (1%)
- Access port problem or tubing leak requiring further surgery
- Nausea/vomiting
- Peptic ulcer disease
- Formation of gallstones due to rapid weight loss

Some of these problems may require further surgical intervention.

Typical Results and Outcomes:

- Following are expected results and outcomes based upon national averages:
- Average weight loss is 45-50% of excess body weight, but with aggressive diet and exercise changes you can lose almost all of your excess weight.
- A weight loss of only about 40% of excess body weight will often show significant improvement in many other medical problems:
    - Many of Type 2 diabetics will get off of medications
    - Hypertensive clients will have improvement or resolution of their hypertension
    - Sleep apnea almost always improves
    - Cholesterol improvement in most clients
    - Arthritic symptoms improve

Laparoscopic Gastric Bypass Surgery

Laparoscopic Roux-en-Y Gastric Bypass was first originated by a group of Bariatric surgeons in California in 1994. This procedure is considered a combination procedure. It works by both restricting the amount of food consumed and also by providing some malabsorption. The surgical outcomes of this procedure seem to indicate that the weight loss results are similar to the traditional "open" procedure as long as the procedures are performed the same way.

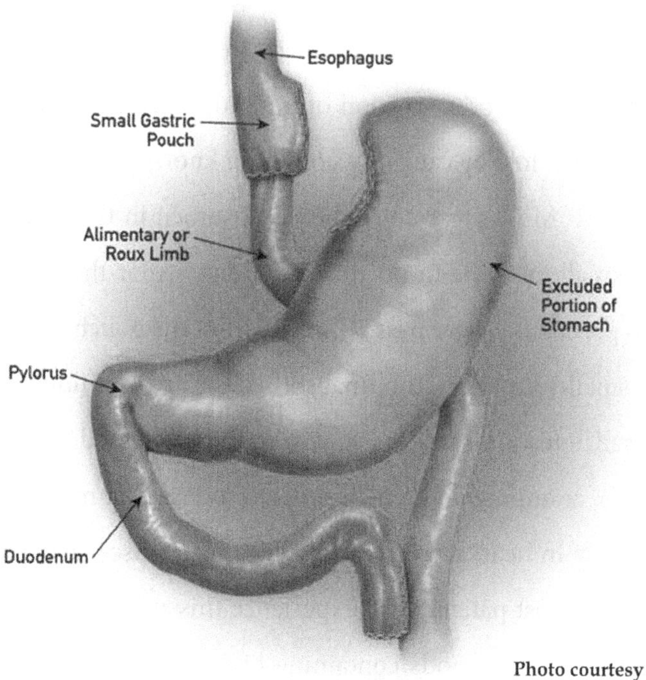

Photo courtesy of
Ethicon Endo-Surgery Inc.

The procedure begins by dividing the stomach to create a "pouch" that limits the amount of food that can be eaten. The pouch is about the size of one's thumb and can hold about 20cc or 2-3 tablespoons of food. The larger excluded stomach, known as the gastric remnant, is stapled closed and separated from the pouch. This portion no longer receives food but has a normal blood supply thereby keeping it healthy.

The second step of the procedure involves taking a portion of the small intestine and creating a "bypass" or "Roux" limb that is connected to the new pouch to provide an outlet for food. This part of the procedure is what creates a slight malabsorption of nutrients to assist in weight loss.

The malabsorptive portion of the procedure also contributes to weight loss by causing a condition known as "Dumping Syndrome". Most sugar consumed is absorbed in the first 1-2 feet of small intestine in normal situations. After the Gastric Bypass procedure sugar passes directly from the pouch into the lower small intestine. The unabsorbed sugar pulls fluid into the small intestine resulting in distension, increased motility (activity), cramping and a neurologic response that may cause an increase in heart rate, sweating, diarrhea, nausea, and even vomiting. Most patients will experience this at least once and will learn to avoid foods containing high sugar content, thus improving the chance for long-term weight loss success.

Risks:

- Possible conversion to an open procedure due to limited access and visibility
- There may be an increased risk for bowel obstruction in the long term
- Death (1:500-1,000)
- Pouch leaks – (1%)
- Deep venous thrombosis (1-2%)
- Pulmonary emboli (1%)
- Abdominal wall hernia (1%)
- Peptic ulcer disease (3-5%)
- Stricture (narrowing) at gastric pouch (1-2%)
- Small bowel obstruction (1-2%)

Typical Results and Outcomes:

The average best weight loss for this procedure is 70% of a client's excess body weight (i.e. if someone is 100 pounds over their ideal body weight, average weight loss outcomes would be 70 pounds).

A weight loss of only about 40% of excess body weight will often show significant improvement in many other medical problems:

- Many Type 2 diabetics will get off of their medications
- Hypertensive clients will have improvement or resolu-

tion of their hypertension

- Sleep apnea almost always improves
- Cholesterol improvement in most clients
- Arthritic symptoms improve

Determining which procedure is right for you will require an evaluation with your surgeon and discussion about your specific situation. As you meet with him/her you will want to find out what their opinion is regarding the preferred weight loss procedure based upon your medical history as well as the number of procedures he/she has performed and their individual outcomes.

CHAPTER 8

Supplemental Bonuses

Action Guide Checklist for Your Ultimate Weight Loss Surgery Success

- Read this book and keep it as a guide throughout your weight loss surgery journey
- Get the videos and pdfs that complement this book at http://www.YourSurgeryPrep.com/

Document your journey as you go and be sure to include your short and long term goals. You will be amazed as you review your progress. It is important to document your physical "numbers" as well as your feelings. Keep track of questions you have for your surgeon and his expert staff of licensed counselors, dieticians, clinical psychologist, insurance coordinator and personal trainers. When they are written down, it is much easier to remember to ask them at your visits.

- Take the time to acknowledge your emotions prior to surgery and after surgery. Discuss them with your surgeon and explore ways to cope with any normal feelings as described in Chapter 2. Support from someone who has already undergone weight loss surgery and/or a clinical psychologist who works regularly with bariatric surgery patients can help you prepare and cope with the many changes that occur with rapid and substantial weight loss.

- Remember that it is ok to put yourself first. Taking care of yourself better prepares you to take care of your loved ones and your ability to function your best in your career.

- Map out your pre-op and post-op schedule. What's written down has a much greater chance of getting done than something left to memory – especially with your busy life. Be sure to attend all of your visits before and after surgery. After surgery, you may be feeling so great you don't need to attend your post-operative visits. Go anyhow! The first year is critical to long term success because sometimes this new tool works "too well". You lose weight easily but if you are not also changing your underlying behaviors, you can be set up for long-term failure. It is imperative to participate in a comprehensive post-operative program. At the Center for Weight Loss Success, we have fine-tuned this process over the past 20 years. All of my patients participate in a comprehensive pre-operative program and post-operative program called Weight Management University for Weight Loss Surgery™. This is a 12 month program that guides you month-by-month through what to expect that month, what to expect the next month, what you should be eating, success stories, recipes, fitness that begins at your level and more. These materials are delivered to their doorstep (written module, DVD and CD) so that by the end of 12 months, they graduate with their "textbook for success". We combine these educational materials with monthly individualized counselings, personal training, fitness classes, educational webinars and weekly Behavior Modification classes accessible live or online for ultimate long-term success. We offer this program for those who visit us on-site as well as those that travel for surgery through the use of online methods in conjunction with the material send to their home. The program is available for anyone having weight loss surgery as well.

- When you eat, think protein first. Sure, right away after surgery hydration is king but adequate amounts of protein along with resistance training exercises (see Chapters 5 & 6) is key to maintaining/building your lean body mass. This is critical to your overall metabolism and your ability to maintain your lower weight for long-term success.

• Know your protein sources. This book shares great protein ideas/sources in Chapter 5. Everyone is different and each day can be different with regards to your taste/tolerance.

• Get moving! The day of surgery you will want to start getting up and moving. Walking is best initially – be sure to follow your surgeons recommendations. I encourage all of my patients to get up and move as soon as possible. It not only helps you physically, but it helps you emotionally as well.

• Don't get discouraged by any plateau's – they are inevitable. Your body wonders why you are losing weight so quickly. As a response, your body will naturally slow down the process and you will hit a plateau. During these times, be sure you are journaling and getting an adequate amount of protein with a controlled carbohydrate count. Increasing your physical activity as well will be the catalyst to pushing you through the plateau and back on track with your weight loss goals.

• Read the rest of this supplemental bonus section. These bonuses are highly regarded by my patients and referred to often…especially the farther they are from the actual date of their surgery.

• Participate actively in a support group. At the Center for Weight Loss Success, we have monthly support group meetings and monthly rewards parties in our nutritional store. The fellowship, stories and support are phenomenal. In addition,

I hold weekly webinars where people get access to additional information. They can suggest topics and have weekly access to me and immediate responses to their questions. Anyone participating in Losing Weight USA (www.losingweightusa.com) can participate as well.

- Share your success with others. Once you get to your goal, it is often hard to hold you back. I have patients who want to hand out our cards to everyone they meet that they feel could benefit. We have an active patient referral program as well. The reality is that it is an individual decision. However, you will be a wealth of knowledge and experience. Even though everyone's journey is a little different, hearing from someone who has been through an experience is immensely helpful. It also helps you to celebrate your success and YOU!
- Finish the rest of this bonus section – you will be glad you did.
- Let us know if you have any questions at success@cfwls.com
- Congratulations!

Weight Loss Surgery Long-Term Success

Making Your Weight Loss "Tool" Most Effective Now...and Later

We want you to succeed now and...forever. Your degree of weight loss and weight maintenance is dependent upon your ability to make Lifestyle/Habit changes including:

1. Proper Use of the Gastric Pouch Tool
2. Adequate Amounts of Activity **AND** Exercise

This section addresses the following:

1. Using Your Small Gastric Pouch for Weight Loss and Weight Maintenance
2. The Return of Hunger
3. Your Ideal Meal Process
4. Principles for Maintaining Satiety
5. Maintaining Your Weight
6. Cottage Cheese Test
7. How to "Beat" the Pouch
8. The five Common Culprits of Poor Weight Loss or Weight Re-Gain

Using Your Stomach Pouch for Weight Loss and Weight Maintenance

Weight loss surgery provides you with a "tool" to help you lose weight and maintain that weight. Just as a craftsman must **learn** how to use a tool and **practice** using that tool for success, learning how to use your stomach pouch/tool will facilitate weight loss and subsequent weight maintenance. This section has been developed to help you learn how to use your pouch/tool. You must **practice** what you **learn** for it to be fully effective.

Stomach (Gastric) Pouch

At the time of your weight loss procedure your gastric pouch is made very small (about 1-2 oz.). The basic mechanism of action of this small gastric pouch is that of **stretch** on the pouch walls after eating a small meal, or even after drinking fluids. This stretch is sensed by nerve receptors on the pouch wall and transmitted to appetite centers at the base of your brain. This produces the feeling of satiety (comfortably satisfied). Ideally you would like this feeling of satiety to be maintained for an extended period of time between meals. Understanding and using your gastric pouch/tool results in better weight loss and subsequent weight maintenance.

As time passes after surgery, you may be concerned that 1.) Your pouch will stretch out and 2.) You will subsequently regain your weight. I will address both of these issues. Yes, your pouch **will** stretch out, but this will **not** necessarily make you regain your weight. The pouch starts out at 1-2 oz. (or even smaller) immediately after surgery. Your pouch will slowly enlarge over time and stabilize at about 2 years. It is difficult to accurately measure the volume of your pouch after surgery. One of the best ways is referred to as the Cottage Cheese Test (CCT - please see separate page). Each person's pouch size will stabilize at a slightly different volume. This may range from 3 - 10 oz. One would suspect that someone who had a "larger" pouch would lose less weight or be more apt to regain weight than someone who has a "smaller" pouch. This is **not** true. People who have a "larger" gastric pouch are just as likely to lose as much weight (and maintain that weight loss) as are those who have a "small" gastric pouch. The reason this occurs is that even the larger gastric pouch (10 oz.) is much smaller than what the normal stomach volume can hold (50-75 oz.).

Then why do some people have more difficulty losing weight and maintaining this weight loss? The reason for this is that success in weight loss after surgery depends not only on having a small gastric pouch but even more on how you **use** your pouch/tool. This means it is extremely important for you to learn how to use the pouch/tool and to put this learning into practice.

The Return of Hunger

Almost all of you will not experience hunger during the first 4-6 months after surgery. Most patients then experience the return of hunger. The "luckiest" few never feel hungry again (This is actually fairly rare).

The reason for the profound satiety (being comfortably satisfied) during the first 4-6 months after surgery is thought to be due to your necessity to drink fluids frequently throughout the day to meet your fluid requirements. Since the gastric pouch is so small during this time, it is probably staying "full" almost all the time and therefore preventing hunger.

Once the gastric pouch enlarges slightly it will then tend to "fill" and "empty". It then takes a little more volume to stimulate the stretch receptors (nerves) on the gastric pouch to give the sensation of satiety. If hunger returns prior to the next meal time, this often means that the gastric pouch is empty. **Water-loading** is the best way for you to alleviate hunger and prevent snacking when this occurs.

Water-loading is for you to drink enough low calorie/no calorie liquid (water is best) to produce the feeling of satiety. This usually takes an amount that is at least twice the volume of your gastric pouch. (Remember that liquids flow through the pouch much more quickly and a larger volume is needed to stimulate the stretch receptors.) The feeling of satiety will last only a short period of time but will help you avoid the need to snack. This can be repeated as often as necessary.

Your Ideal Meal Process

- Do not skip meals
- There should be about 5 hours between meals – a **planned** snack is permitted and should be protein and/or fiber based
- Optimal meal - more solid type foods such as finely cut meat and minimally cooked vegetables and salads
- Take meals over 15-20 minutes (i.e. a shorter period of time than what we recommend right after surgery)
- Do not drink liquids until 45-60 minutes **following** the meal
- After 1 ½ - 2 hours, begin drinking low or no calories liquids somewhat **slowly** (to avoid "dumping")
- Progressively accelerate drinking up to 15 minutes before the next meal (stopping drinking 15 minutes prior to meals allows the pouch to empty of liquids so that you start with an empty stomach when you eat)
- Water-loading in the 2 hours prior to eating will help

avoid a significant thirst response.

- Water loading can be done any time in the 2-3 hours preceding a meal if hunger is experienced.

Principles for Maintaining Satiety

- The pouch needs to be filled with adequate wall distension with each meal (i.e. no snacking or "grazing").
- Keep the pouch filled over time and slow down the emptying time by eating solid foods and avoiding liquids for 15 minutes before and 45-60 minutes after eating. **This is the most important lifestyle change after weight loss surgery.**
- Eat adequate protein with each meal. Think protein first.
- The **enemy** is **high calorie liquids and high carbohydrate foods.**
- It is not necessary to follow every rule all the time. It is all right to break the rules once in a while. The important thing is to be aware that you are breaking the rules and **not** to make a habit of it.

Maintaining Your Weight

Weight control is the result of satiety (comfortably satisfied), or the absence of abnormal hunger associated with the ingestion of the number of calories sufficient to meet your metabolic needs. [Weight will remain stable if calories ingested (food) = calories used (activity)].

You have worked hard to lose the excess weight, but now a few extra pounds are beginning to creep back on. When weight begins to increase many people's first response is "*There's something wrong with my surgery!*". Although this is not impossible, it is actually fairly rare. In the majority, this "failure" often represents the inability to maintain post meal satiety long enough to prevent snacking before the next meal time. (Please review the Ideal Meal Process and Principles for Maintaining Satiety above.)

Remember that this is a **lifelong** commitment. It can be a very difficult journey. Help is available through your bariatric surgeon's office, their support group and their professional team of dieticians, counselors, and many others depending on your individual circumstances. In addition, you can find specialized help with diet, behavior modification and fitness at the Center for Weight Loss Success (www.cfwls.com, success@cfwls.com or 757-873-1880).

Cottage Cheese Test

- The Cottage Cheese Test (CCT) is used to estimate gastric pouch size.
- Fast for about 1 hour prior to the test to make sure that the pouch is empty.
- Do this test at a meal which is your "prime time" for best appetite.
- For those of you who despise cottage cheese, you may substitute thick oatmeal.
- For best results, do this test 3-4 times over a 1 week period and average the results.

Test:

- Eat from a standard carton of cottage cheese until comfortably satisfied, taking **no longer** than **5 minutes** to complete the meal.
- Fill the resulting space in the cottage cheese carton with milk or water.
- Pour off the liquid and measure it to the nearest ½ oz.
- The amount of cottage cheese eaten is a relatively good estimate of your stomach pouch size

How to "Beat" the Pouch

I do **not** recommend that you do this, but if you find that you are having difficulty losing weight (or maintaining weight after your weight has stabilized) then review these. See if any apply to your situation. These are all common reasons that will **stop weight loss** and possibly **begin weight regain.**

1. Liquid/soft high calorie meals
2. High calorie liquids between meals
3. Frequent meals or grazing
4. Eating a meal over 30-45 minutes
5. Drinking liquids with meals to enhance gastric pouch emptying
6. Taking liquids shortly after eating to increase gastric pouch emptying and decrease the satiety period
7. Eating crispy carbohydrates such as chips, crackers, popcorn etc.
8. NOT exercising

You should <u>not</u> be doing these things
unless you want to regain your weight!!!!!!!

Five Common Culprits of Poor Weight Loss or Weight Re-Gain

If you are frustrated with poor/slower weight loss or eventual weight re-gain, we can commonly track it back to one of these five culprits.

1. **Depression** – Emotional health is as important as physical health. Although depression is not a problem for most after surgery, it can be a significant deterrent to optimal weight loss. It is important to identify depression (admit that it is ok) and seek appropriate treatment so you can move on with your weight loss journey.

2. **Not Exercising** – We require each of you to complete a fitness evaluation with a personal trainer which is included with the program. The reason for this is because we believe some form of consistent exercise is essential for optimal success. You should determine what form of exercise is right for you and begin your exercise plan before surgery. We cannot over-emphasize the importance of this factor. Although most find it difficult to begin an exercise plan, those that take that plunge never regret it. It can only enhance your weight loss experience and progress.

3. **Drinking High Calorie Liquids** – Many do not realize the excessive amount of sugar and calories contained in

some liquids (i.e. Gatorade, Juice, Soda). As a result, you may "waste" calories on such liquids. This can significantly impede your weight loss. It is better to choose water, water with lemon, Fruit2O, Crystal Light or other low or no calorie drink options.

4. "Grazing" – After the first 2 months or so, you should have progressed to three meals per day with some higher protein snacks in between. If not, you may develop the habit of "grazing" or eating throughout the day. If this is the case, you tend to take in a significantly higher amount of calories throughout the day (more than what your body needs). This will slow down your weight loss and can potentially cause weight re-gain. Please guard yourself against such habits and be sure to follow the section "utilizing the small gastric pouch for weight loss and weight maintenance" earlier in this section.

5. Eating and Drinking at the Same Time – When you eat and drink at the same time, the food is "washed through" the stomach quickly. It is important to hydrate yourself by drinking a low/no calorie beverage approximately 30 minutes prior to eating. In this way, your hunger will be decreased. When you eat, you should not drink at the same time. As a result, your "pouch" will remain fuller for a longer period of time. Thus, you will remain satisfied for a longer period of time. Be sure to stop eating before you truly feel "full". It is a slow communication process from your stomach to your brain that indicates a feeling of fullness. Thus, you may overeat and realize it too late. This can be a very uncomfortable feeling.

Keys to Successful Weight Loss and Long-Term Weight Control

Try to make these "keys" Habits for Life

Eating - Don't skip meals. Food choices should be low fat and low sugar. Think "Protein First". Eating should be approached as "how little can I eat and be satisfied", NOT "how much can I cram in there".

Drinking – Try to avoid drinking with your meals. Beverages should be non-caloric and non-carbonated. Drinking 8 glasses of water each day is a good idea with any weight loss plan.

Vitamins – Multivitamins should be taken daily – ***Forever.*** Other vitamins and/or supplements may be needed depending upon individual needs.

Sleeping – Make sure you are well rested. The most successful patients sleep an average of 7 hours each night.

Exercise – Regular exercise is ***extremely*** important and should be done ***at least*** 3-4 times per week for at least 30-40 minutes.

Personal Responsibility – Successful patients take personal responsibility for weight loss/weight control. *It's up to you!!* No one else can lose the weight for you. The surgery is only a "tool". ***You*** have to use this tool appropriately.

Informative Websites

Center for Weight Loss Success, PC

Dr. Clark's Center for Weight Loss Success provides a comprehensive surgical and medical weight loss program including all of the components necessary for long-term success (medically supervised, individualized eating plans, lifestyle/habit modification classes, fitness classes and personal training). The staff is specifically trained to assist weight loss surgery patients. Visit our main site at www.cfwls.com for more information.

1. Follow us on Facebook – helpful posts and support each and every day along with contests, discounts, supportive stories and more!

- Go to http://www.facebook.com/weightlossdrclark

or just go to www.cfwls.com and click on the Facebook icon in the upper right hand corner.

- If you already have a Facebook account, log in from

this webpage (at the top). If you haven't already, you will want to "like" our page and share it with all of your friends on Facebook who want to lose weight so they can become a fan too!

- If you do not have a Facebook account, you can just go to this page every day to see our tips or to receive them automatically, sign up for a free Facebook account from this page and then click on the box "like" once your account is active.

2. Did you know Dr. Clark has a You Tube channel where you can view hundreds of his helpful short videos? Go to http://www.youtube.com/docweightloss today! Video is a fun and easy way to see testimonials and his helpful tips on how to lose weight!

3. Dr. Clark also provides valuable information about weight loss through his blog at www.cfwls.com/blog.

4. Sign up for Dr. Clark's free weekly podcast series at www.cfwls.com/podcasts. You can listen to new information about weight loss weekly on the go wherever you are such as in your car, at the gym or on a walk around the neighborhood or local park.

5. Follow Dr. Clark on Twitter: (http://www.twitter.com/docweightloss).

Follow what Dr. Clark is doing – better yet, get it right

on your phone by text messaging "follow docweightloss" to 40404.

6. Sign up for our ongoing Weight Loss Membership Program called Losing Weight USA (www.LosingWeightUSA.com) to help with all of your weight loss efforts.

7. Tune into our online TV channel at www.docweightloss.tv for up-to-date coverage on weight loss surgery and other pertinent weight loss news/information

8. Nutrition Data -This website is useful in finding the nutritional content of all foods and some common restaurants. www.nutritiondata.com

9. These websites are useful for both nutritional and exercise information. www.fitday.com and www.myfitnesspal.com

Index

[1] http://www.wvdhhr.org/bph/oehp/obesity/mortality.htm

[2] Lemonick, M.D. The Power of Mood, Time Magazine, p. 68-69.

Made in the USA
Monee, IL
14 September 2026

62974517R00098